Portion Perfection
for Bariatrics:
International Edition

First published 2014. Revised and updated 2022.
© Great Ideas In Nutrition 2014-2022, Phone +61 7 5599 2082, Australia.

Author: Clark, Amanda, 1964-
Title: Portion Perfection for Bariatrics: International Edition / Amanda Clark
Edition: 1st Edition
ISBN: 978-0-9925043-2-8 (pbk.)
Subjects: Cookery. Low-fat diet-Recipes. Health. Nutrition. Bariatric Surgery
Dewey Number: 641.563
Published by: Great Ideas in Nutrition – www.greatideas.net.au
Editor: Anna Crago
Design: Simone Young – www.tweedcoastgraphicdesign.com.au
Photography: Enigma Visions, Brett Backhouse and Brodie Clark
Food Styling: Lloyd Hanger
Nutrition Assistant: Anna Millichamp
Printed by Classic Print, Singapore

Disclaimers

While all care has been taken in the preparation of this book and every effort has been made to represent product details correctly, no responsibility is accepted for any errors, omissions or inaccuracies, or for any representation whether expressed or implied, which is beyond the control of the author/publisher. Foods represented in this book are as per generally available brands. Some estimates have been made.

Not every food that meets the criteria is represented in this book and it would not be practical/feasible to do so. The book is intended as a guide rather than an exhaustive listing of all foods which meet the criteria. The appearance of a food or product in the book is at the discretion of the author and is not guaranteed even if it meets all criteria. No fee has been paid/received in return for any reference to a product in the book.

Further, the criteria for inclusion/determination of everyday or occasional foods have been set with reference to various sources of existing criteria and the author's own professional judgement. Criteria may change based on current nutritional knowledge or research. Glycemic index (GI) is considered to be an important factor in selecting appropriate products for weight control. Not all products have been measured for GI. Therefore some professional discretion has been exercised based on the author's experience and no correspondence will be entered into.

Calories shown may be approximations and rounded to the nearest 100 Calories for ease of calculations. Also, breakfast cereal volumes have been rounded to the nearest ¼ cup. Protein contents have been rounded to the nearest gram.

This book is intended to be used as a general reference. It is a general guide only and does not constitute advice on individual or particular circumstances, or a substitute for the advice of a health care professional on any specific health issue/condition. It is recommended that a dietitian or health care professional be consulted to check that a weight loss plan is suitable and that specific advice be sought in relation to any specific health issues/conditions. The author/publisher accepts no responsibility for any failure to seek or follow the advice of a health care professional and will not be liable for such failure. Every effort is made to represent products accurately. No responsibility is taken for errors or omissions.

Portion Perfection
for Bariatrics:
International Edition

by Amanda Clark Adv APD

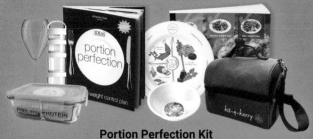
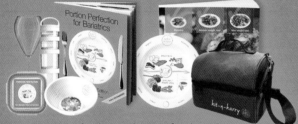

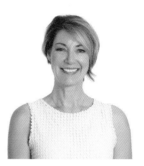

About the Author

Amanda Clark is an Advanced Accredited Practising Dietitian (Adv APD), and a leader within her field. She is known for making scientific concepts easy to understand, and in 2006 Amanda received the prestigious Dietitian's Association of Australia's President's Award for Innovation.

She completed a bachelor degree in biochemistry and human physiology from Macquarie University and postgraduate qualifications in Nutrition and Dietetics at the University of Sydney. Amanda has 25 years experience and runs her own successful Gold Coast-based practice, Great Ideas in Nutrition, which specialises in delivering clear, concise and realistic advice about food and nutrition. Amanda also runs an online nutrition resource shop, stocking practical and trusted books and resources.

She lives on the Gold Coast and is married with two sons.

Acknowledgements

Thank you so much to all my lovely client-friends who have contributed to my level of expertise. Thank you for the positive feedback on things that worked and guidance on the things that didn't. Particularly Cath, Cathey, Deb, Esther and Vicki. I owe some of my expertise to your inspirational commitment.

To my family: Ray, Aimon and Brodie Clark, and Jan and Ken Railton.

My staff: Jenny Lahiff, Carolyn Rosenberg, Alesha Soanes, Carly Barlow and Selina Howard.

My project team: Simone Young, Brodie Clark, Nordeen Chakroune.

My mentors and experts: Dr Paul Anderson, Mr Krishna Epari, A/prof John Dixon, Dr Candice Silverman, Pennie Taylor. Also Dr Cathryn Murphy, Donna Mitchell and Colleen Cook.

My international colleagues and with particular mention of Stacy Paine, Brenda Hoenh, Dr Laure Demattia, Megan Tomczyszyn and Sukwan Jolley.

I haven't had bariatric surgery so what would I know?

I am merely a lateral thinker who can put all my knowledge of food and nutrition and my experience in weight control and food management - both personal and professional - into a concept that makes sense. I hope you find it useful.

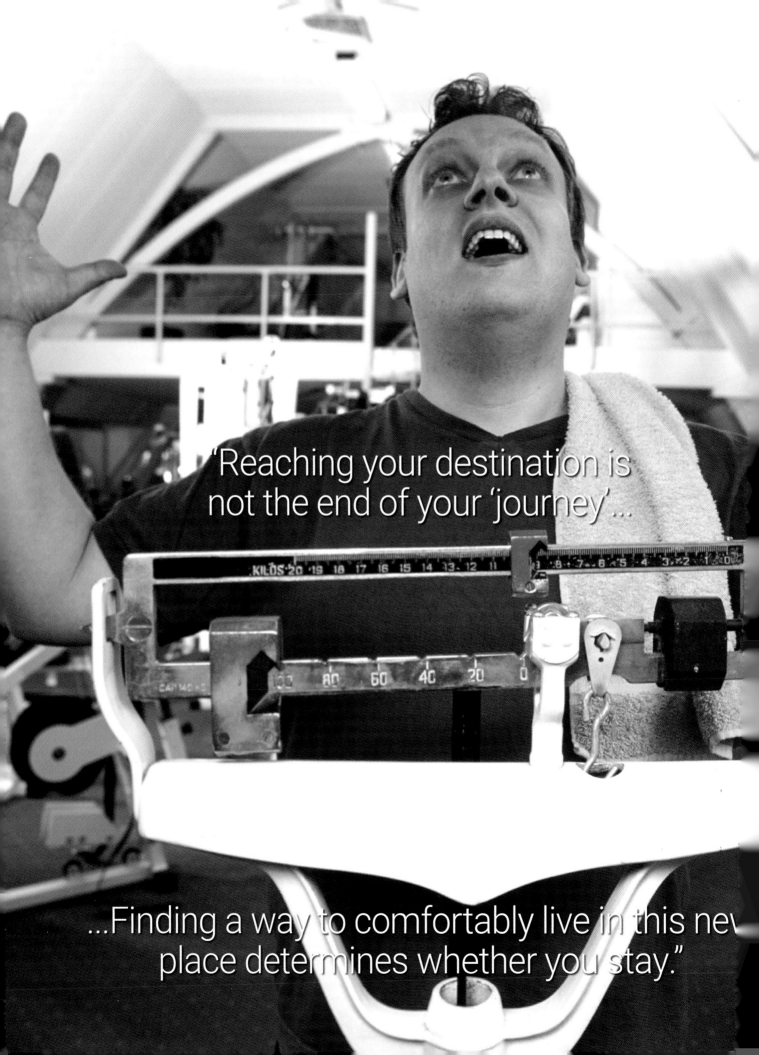

Foreword by Dr Candice Silverman

As a surgeon who runs a high-volume bariatric surgery program, I have had the pleasure and good fortune of working closely with Amanda Clark for almost a decade. Amanda has over 25 years of clinical experience and is renowned nationally and internationally for her work with bariatric surgery patients.

Obesity is largely a genetic disease, and in severe cases the most effective treatment is surgery. Surgery can reverse the diseases that are caused by excess weight such as diabetes, which is why it is also called "metabolic surgery".

People who have had a bariatric procedure need to make adjustments to the food they eat to manage their changed alimentary tract after surgery, therefore nutritional advice provided by Amanda to my patients is imperative for their weight loss success and overall health.

To assist people who have had surgery, Amanda has developed a beautifully illustrated, factual, practical, flexible way to guide healthy eating. What does healthy eating after bariatric surgery look like? This book provides excellent information on not only what it looks like but what this feels like, tastes like and smells like. I personally ensure all my bariatric surgery patients receive a copy of this book, *Portion Perfection for Bariatrics*. I highly recommend this book to anyone considering bariatric surgery, as an invaluable resource to assist with successful weight loss and weight maintenance.

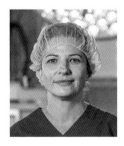 **Dr Candice Silverman** is a general surgeon who specialises in bariatric surgery. She has a passion for robotic surgery and is the leading robotic bariatric surgeon in Australia. She believes in a multi-disciplinary approach to provide the best care for her patients.

Client input from bariatric surgery recipients

I owe much of my expertise to the education I have received from band, sleeve and bypass owners. I have invited comment along the way from a range of consumers.

Kim Hamilton – Bypass Recipient

All my adult life I have struggled with my weight. It was the stereotypical yoyo - I would lose weight and then regain plus some, and this continued for forty years.

I have always tried to be active, even at my highest weight of 245 pounds / 111kg. If I exercised in the morning though, I was exhausted for the rest of the day. Everything was an effort. I noticed that I didn't have the confidence in myself to do things I'd always wanted to do because of my weight.

At the age of 57 I came to the conclusion that I needed to consider bariatric surgery to improve my quality of life. I had been trying to lose weight for most of my adult life. I tried all sorts of products and exercise but I would always regain the weight.

I started to research what was involved with bariatric surgery and the different options available. My family and close friends were very supportive of my decision, so I took the giant leap and made an appointment to talk to a surgeon and moved forward with gastric bypass surgery in September 2016. The surgeon also explained working with dietitians and psychologists throughout the process is a very important step for a positive outcome.

My dietitian introduced me to Portion Perfection, which I found to be an amazing set of tools. I found that the visual reference helped to lock information in my mind easier. The bowl and bariatric plate are extremely helpful and five years later, I am still using them. I find the Snacker very handy and the guidance for quantity and food examples. It's perfect for taking snacks with you if you're going shopping, to work or to the beach.

I am currently 167 pounds / 76kg. Since losing my weight, I feel healthier, fitter and happier and am enjoying life. I now have the confidence to do those things I've always wanted to.

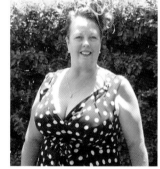 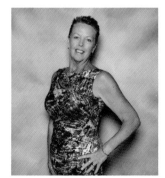

Before   **After**

John Roehrig – Sleeve Owner

I am a Type 2 diabetic and have been for half my life, it was diabetes that drove me to seek bariatric surgery. I had been on the roller coaster ride of losing weight through exercise then ballooning back to bigger than before. When my weight was down, my diabetic control was excellent and required little or no medication.

Just when things were going well, I would become complacent and eventually I would regain the weight and revert to poor blood sugar control. I started medication, which I thought would be the answer, but my weight and medication kept increasing until I was injecting insulin 4 times a day.

In 2018 I visited friends in Japan, and it was then I really confronted my problem. I couldn't enjoy myself and was in constant fear of having hypos. My weight had increased to over 265lb / 120 kg, my mobility was poor, and I felt a burden on the group of friends I was travelling with.

During my next check up, my doctor suggested gastric sleeve surgery. I went through the process with the surgeon, psychologist and dietitian and I had my surgery.

As I progressively lost weight under the program, I found myself with more energy and I undertook an exercise routine which helped even more. I still maintain consistent exercise, and this has enabled me to maintain my weight around 187lb / 85 kg. I am feeling the best I have for many a year. I am no longer using insulin or taking blood pressure medication.

The portion control plates and dishes have been a great help, enabling me to visualize how much I need, not want.

I have come to understand that sustained loss of weight is a combination of making the right food choices, monitoring the amount you consume and exercise. My advice for anyone considering bariatric surgery would be that they also need to make lifestyle changes. The surgery will help lose the weight, but good dietary control will help maintain the loss.

This book, and the Portion Perfection system is an important component in maintaining good health and enjoying the lifestyle that accompanies this.

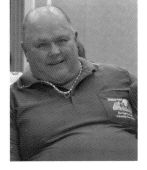

Before

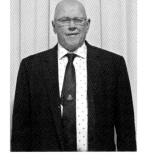

After

Colleen Cook – Bypass Patient

I quietly and secretly investigated weight loss surgery many years ago in 1993. I had a personal consultation with a surgeon and knew that this was the answer for me. Unfortunately, my insurance would not cover it and paying cash was not a possibility at that time.

So, I just kept it to myself and thought, "Someday, some way I will do this." Years passed and I reached my all-time heavy weight of 250 pounds (116kg). At 5'2" (157cm), I was unhappy and unhealthy, but still my insurance wouldn't cover it. On Thanksgiving weekend of 1995, my wonderful husband, knowing of my unhappiness and my deteriorating health, suggested that we take a second mortgage on our home and use the equity to pay cash for this surgery. Some of my friends were buying new cars and new furniture; I got a new body (and now I have the new car and the new furniture)! It was certainly a risk to undergo major surgery uninsured, but it was a risk we were willing to take. The decision to have weight-loss surgery has proven to be one of the best decisions I have ever made. It has been worth every penny.

As a successful weight loss surgery patient, I have also had the wonderful privilege to work within the bariatric community since 1998. I am the author of the bariatric best seller, The Success Habits of Weight loss Surgery Patients and President of Bariatric Support Centers International.

I was honoured to meet Amanda Clark on a trip to Australia in 2012 and continue to be impressed with her work and important contribution. This book, Portion Perfection is an outstanding real-world resource filled with wonderful tips and ideas designed to help weight loss surgery patients plan and prepare healthy, balanced and perfectly portioned meals.

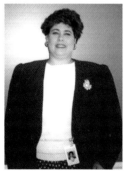

Before   **After**

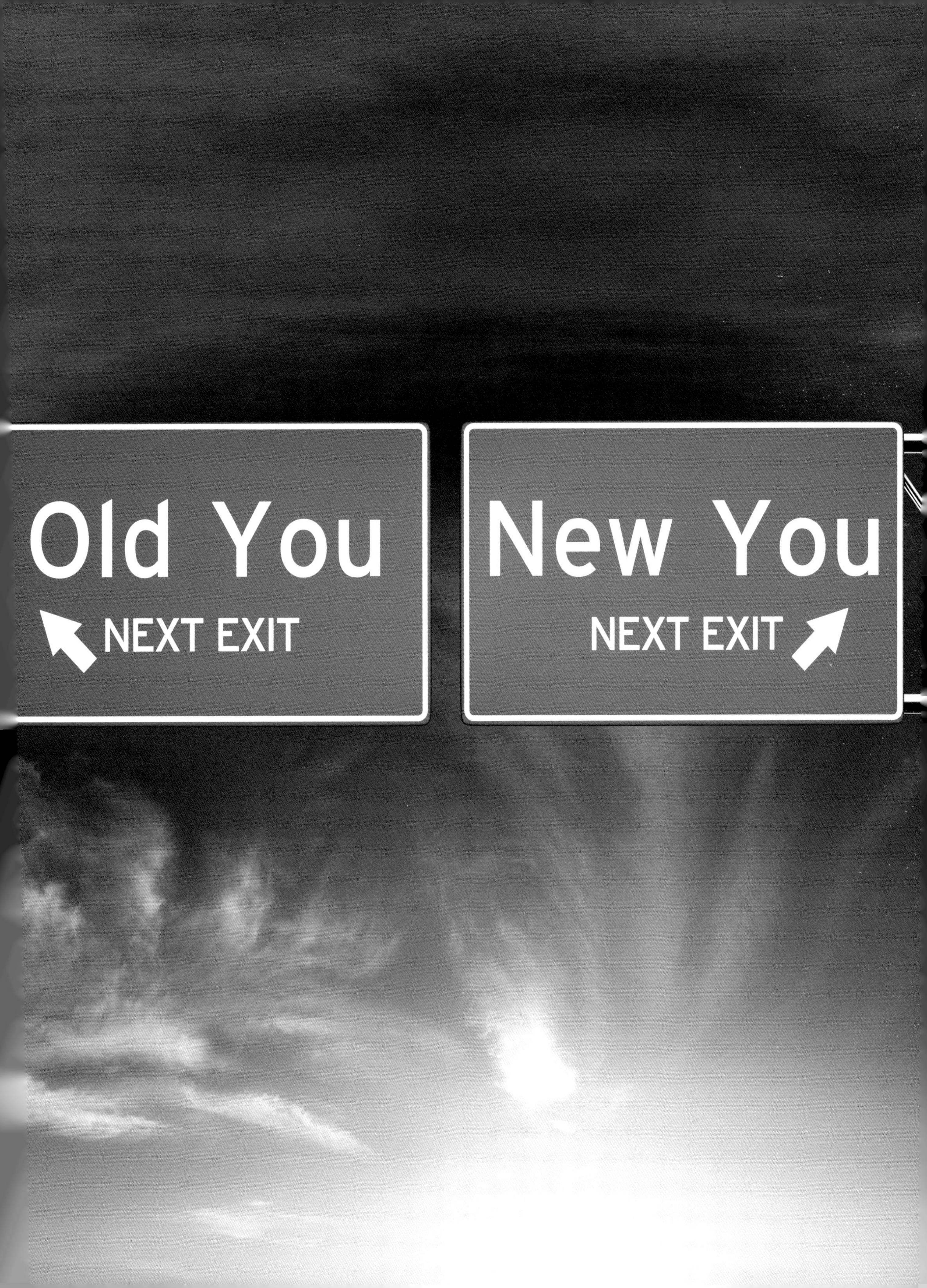
Old You
NEXT EXIT
New You
NEXT EXIT

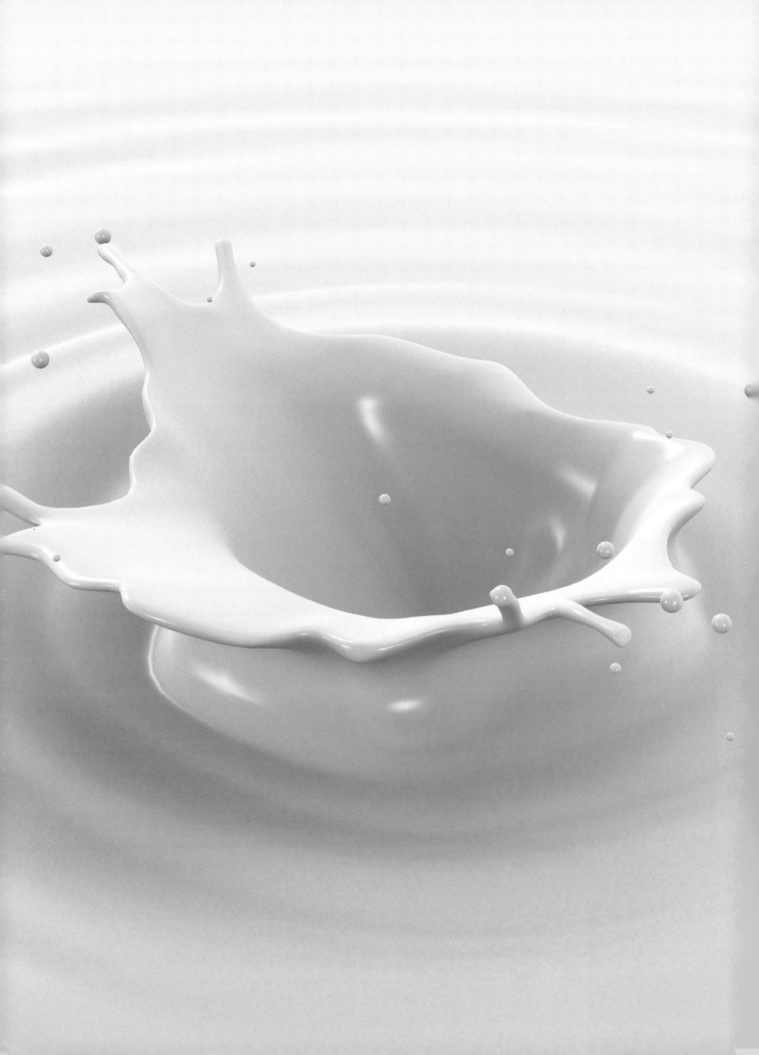

Contents

Introduction   15

Chapter 1:   Portion Problems Around the World   19

Chapter 2:   The Portion Perfection Concept   27

Chapter 3:   Nutritional Considerations   35

Chapter 4:   Portion Perfection in Practice   45

Chapter 5:   Food Guide Basics   54

Chapter 6:   Breakfast   57

Chapter 7:   Lunch   71

Chapter 8:   Dinner   85

Chapter 9:   Snacks   93

Chapter 10:   Appendices   111

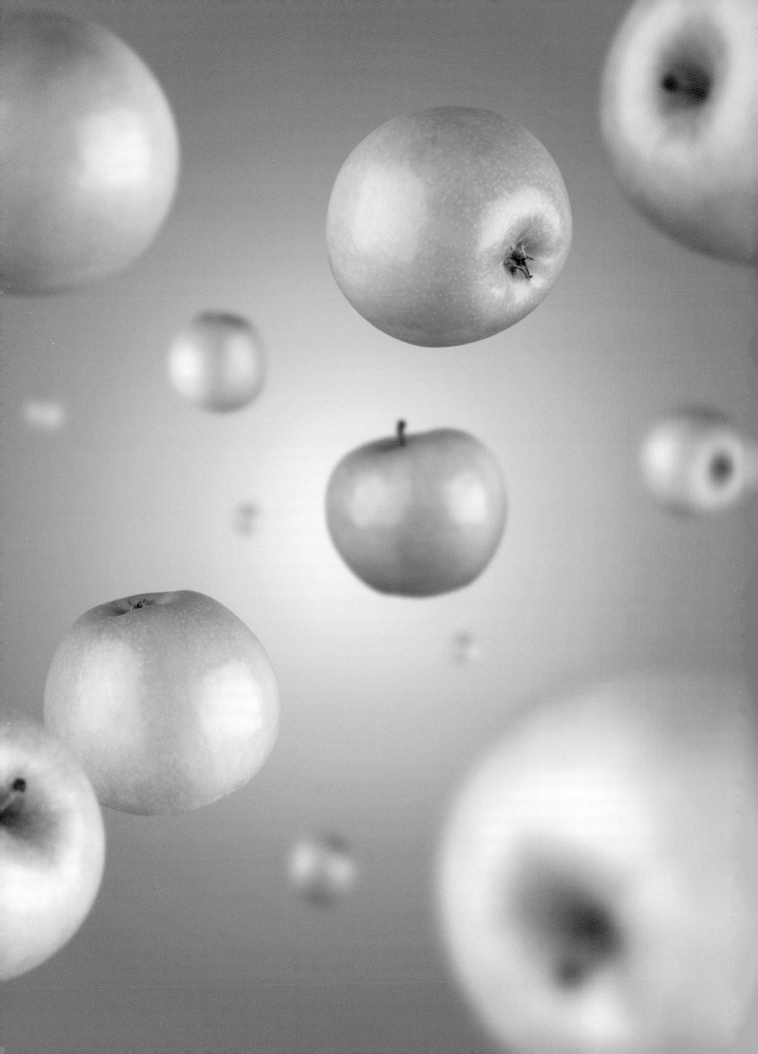

Introduction

In my 25 plus years of practise as a dietitian, one of my major priorities has been to make dietary concepts simple and understandable for my clients. I developed the Portion Perfection Plate for just that purpose. The Portion Perfection Plate is a dinner plate with ideal portion size and nutritional balance guides printed on it so that you can quickly and easily monitor the amount and type of food you serve.

The Portion Perfection Bowl soon followed. This bowl is used for monitoring portion sizes of soups, purees, cereals and desserts. These products can be purchased online at www.portiondiet.com or www.amazon.com/portionperfection.

Around this time, I published *Portion Perfection: a visual weight control plan*. This book can be used in conjunction with the Portion Perfection Plate and Bowl. Its aim is to help guide weight control food choices for the entire day. I've found that many people zone out when presented with a list of dietary options – but that they respond well to visual images, and so I often use pictures rather than words with my clients.

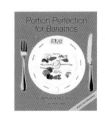

The plate and bowl concept is an effective way to monitor your progress on an ongoing basis, and the standard (purple) version of *Portion Perfection - a visual weight control plan* and all the associated tools can be used by the whole family.

It was following the success and positive feedback from the initial plate that the Portion Perfection Bariatric Plate was developed. This plate was specifically designed for those who have undergone sleeve gastrectomy, any form of gastric bypass or gastric banding. This book, *Portion Perfection for Bariatrics*, forms the basis for the range of bariatric Portion Perfection tools.

Portion Perfection for Bariatrics includes photographs of the ideal portion size for bariatric surgery recipients during the weight loss phase. It is assumed that you have completed your post-surgery regime which may include fluids and puree and you are ready for solid food.

The Portion Perfection range includes, recipe guides that perfectly fit the concept, lunch containers, snack containers, wine glasses and more. They serve to influence the amount you usually eat or drink without having to count calories or measure foods externally.

It is not my goal to educate on the surgery or to replace existing resources designed for bariatric surgery patients, nor the advice of your team. It is my intention to lend my own interpretation to help clarify what to do, what to buy and how much to serve.

It's easy to lose perspective when it comes to knowing how much to eat. Did you know that restaurant, take away and packaged food portions, not to mention dinner plates and bowls, have been getting steadily bigger over the years? External factors like this certainly don't help us with our nutritional decision-making. In this book I hope to give some answers to all those who have lost perspective when it comes to the question of *how much should I eat?*

Stomachs are stretchy membranes. Some people can fit two pizzas comfortably whilst others are happy on half a sandwich. It's all to do with the stretch!

The value of any bariatric surgery is that you effectively have a whole new stomach and an opportunity to maintain a tiny appetite. The problem is that if you've been a two-pizza eater, you've stretched your stomach before and you could do it again. That's where portion control comes in. Every time you eat past the point of satisfaction, and move on to fullness, the first thing that happens is your stomach stretches to capacity and the second thing that happens is you regurgitate food. It's vitally important to the long-term effectiveness of your procedure for you to listen for that moment of satisfaction. If you regularly fill your stomach to 'fullness', you will gradually increase the capacity of your new stomach and dull the sensation of satisfaction.

Portion Perfection for Bariatrics shows you the ideal portion sizes of common foods. This information will help you to protect your new stomach volume. Eating the right amount – and knowing the consequences of eating too much – will become truly simple.

I have found that the Portion Perfection concept helps both overeaters and undereaters, as well as those with serious eating disorders. It's also useful for those just wishing to be healthier and to eat better-balanced meals.

I would also like to influence processed food manufacturers to take a look at the serving sizes they offer the market. We are the customers, and if we let the market know that we want snacks in 100 Cal (420 kJ) serves, that is what we will get – eventually. Why not start the process at your local supermarket by purchasing the portion sizes shown in this book?

Portion Perfection for Bariatrics will help you see through the ever-increasing portion sizes all around you. These portion sizes – and their effect on your body – are probably in part behind your decision to undergo weight loss surgery. The division between everyday, vital and occasional foods will help identify the right foods for you and point you towards good nutrition. And, importantly, seeing what the right serve looks like for weight loss really can help keep you on track.

This book is aimed at everyone around the world who has undergone sleeve gastrectomy, gastric bypass or gastric banding with the aim of achieving and maintaining their ideal body weight.

Chapter 1 sets out the context of portion control, and explains how as a society we've lost our way when it comes to how much to eat. Chapter 2 introduces the tools, and the Portion Perfection concept, more thoroughly. In Chapter 3, you'll learn about some underlying nutritional considerations. Chapter 4 leads you through the practical considerations in using the Portion Perfection tools. Finally, Chapter 5 provides you with a pictorial guide to food portions for many common foods and meals.

Portion Perfection for Bariatrics should provide you with the tools and information you need to eat healthy, controlled portions.

I hope you find the book, plate, bowl, and all the tools useful so that you may turn your attention to other things in life and stop worrying about your weight. I welcome feedback on your experiences - please contact me via any method below.

Amanda Clark

E: info@portiondiet.com

Facebook page: portionperfection

Facebook group: bariatricsurgeryeating

Instagram: portionperfection

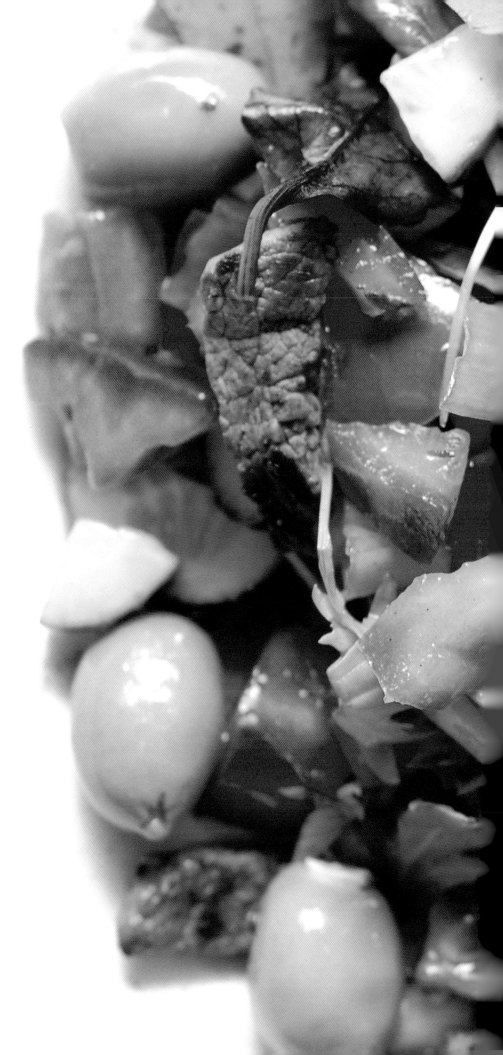

"The bigger
the plate,
the more
we eat."

Chapter 1:
Portion Problems Around the World

Recent data from the United States, Europe and Australia show that we are eating up to 500 Cals / 2100 kJ per day more than we did 20 or 30 years ago.

Experts agree that:

- We are eating more without being aware of it.

- Marketing encourages us to eat large servings of high-Calorie foods, and

- Advertising encourages us to eat more often, and suggests that it's normal to eat less healthy foods all the time, or at every meal.

It's also true that we generally do less exercise these days than we used to. And, of course, less exercise also contributes to the amount of food that we store as body fat.

The latest global estimates suggest that an additional 1,200,000,000 (1.2 billion) people will be overweight or obese by 2030, with the greatest proportion of those new qualifiers being residents of the UK, USA or Australia. The level of diabetes will likely follow and this is suspiciously in line with an ongoing increase in the Calorie content of many common food serves.

So many people are searching for the foods they can eat to sustain a healthy weight. Every year we're enticed by a new fad diet or the 'discovery' of a new diet secret or superfood. The more pertinent question, though, is to determine *how much is the right amount of food to eat to achieve and maintain a healthy weight* and then let's modify eating patterns and portions to equate to this.

What we eat is certainly a problem for some, but *how much* we eat is becoming a problem for all of us.

We fear for the future of our children, and quite rightly so. The fact is that we have probably reached our maximum life expectancy potential, and even with the best medical care, our children may live a shorter life than ourselves.

Think Calories

We've shown both Calories and kilojoules in most areas of the book. Australia uses kilojoules as their correct metric measurement, but we find in practice that Calories are much smaller numbers, which are easier to add and multiply! So if you don't speak either language, start learning to think Calories to stay on track.

1 Calorie = approx 4.2 kJ, so roughly multiplying or dividing by 4 will convert Calories to kilojoules or vice versa.

What can be done to remedy the situation?

Gastric restrictive surgeries such as sleeve gastrectomy, gastric bypass and gastric banding work because they result in satisfaction from smaller portions of food. The size of the stomach does nothing magical to make body fat disappear immediately, but it does influence how much you feel like eating, and that's where you come in. It's your job to keep portion sizes small by stopping when you sense that new feeling of 'satisfaction' and exercise to help your body to stay healthy as it transforms.

The reason it was hard to lose weight before the surgery is that the body is defending it's fat. We have a myriad of hormones that influence our appetite. They all have very chemical names but one, (Grhelin) is produced by the stomach when it is empty to prompt us to eat, others are produced at either the beginning or the end of the small intestine to tell the brain that food has made it there. One, (Leptin) is produced by the fat stores themselves to message whether their stockpile is depleting and others (including Insulin) are released in response to nutrients arriving in the bloodstream. All this information goes to the brain via the blood supply or a major nerve, where it decides whether to prompt us to eat or not.

There are a few modern day problems which interfere with this previously effective system.

1. There are chemicals appearing in our food, our cosmetics, our cleaning products and our environment which have been termed "obesogens". These chemicals impersonate or override some of those natural signals to distort the messages and result in the drive to eat more or conserve energy by resting.

2. Our own bodies and the bacteria within them are producing hormones related to stress or lack of sleep that interfere with the natural system and also send us in search of food.

3. Food marketing and increasing portion sizes unconsciously influence how much we eat, and it only takes a few extra bites each meal to result in significant weight gain over a year.

4. The thin ideal pushed by TV, advertising and social media popularizes stringent diets aiming for rapid weight loss. This makes those hormones kick in to eventually make us even hungrier, less active and enables our bodies to function on less food resulting in those fat stores filling back up.

How does bariatric surgery help?

In bariatric surgery, some of the chemical signaling is changed. The effect is very strong initially and then some components of this wear off over time.

Almost all current bariatric surgeries include a component of reducing the size of the stomach. Nerves sense the tension in the stomach wall, and with a small stomach it doesn't take much food to initiate a satisfaction or fullness message.

Bypass surgeries result in food arriving further down in your intestine sooner, triggering early release of hormones there which also reduce the drive to eat.

These higher levels of hormones are also thought to spill over into your saliva resulting in altered taste perception. Many people recognize this as sweet foods not tasting as good as they previously did.

Over time though, bodies adapt to the modified hormone levels and sweet foods start to taste the way they used to. This is why it is important to have made changes to your lifestyle and the food you have at home if sugar has been a problem for you in the past. Create new habits that don't significantly involve sugar and keep problem food and drinks out of the house where possible.

So what can we do?

We need to establish a healthy lifestyle that we can live with longterm. Year one after surgery is the absolute best time to establish this whilst you are not bothered by appetite, but it's never too late to change.

Changing habits is always difficult because our brains tend to guide us along the paths we have travelled before. To make new pathways we need to carry out new behaviours repeatedly.

It's really helpful to follow a system of eating less that defines behavior and creates routines or patterns your brain can catch on to.

First, let's explore one of the major triggers to eating more than we need – portion size.

How did we come to be eating so much?

I believe that clever marketing and eating too much have left us dazed and confused about how much we actually need to eat. Here's some examples from my home, that I'm sure you can relate to.

A meal for weight maintenance ideally contains 450–550 Calories (Cals) / 1890-2310 Kilojoules, and a snack 200 Cals / 840kJ.

Chocolate bars

Think back about 20 years ago, if you can! Can you remember how big chocolate bars were? Strangely, they were much smaller than they are today. For example, look at what's happened to the Kit Kat, which was one of the smallest bars on the market 20 years ago. Today, that very same snack is one of the largest on the market.

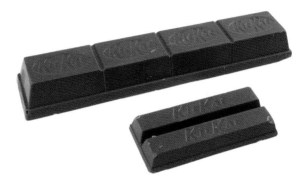

20 years ago:
100 Cals / 420 kJ
Today:
409 Cals / 1717 kJ

Originally Kit Kats were 0.7 oz / **20 g** (around 100 Cals / **420 kJ**), but now there's the Kit Kat Chunky King Size which is 2.75 oz / **78 g** (409 Cals / **1717 kJ**). It's gone from an acceptable snack to almost a meal's worth of Calories!

Let's look at some more comparisons between portion sizes 20 years ago and those today.

Take-away coffees

Twenty years ago, a take-away coffee would have come in a 7 fl oz / **200 ml** polystyrofoam cup. It would have been made on water, and even if you added full cream milk and sugar, it wouldn't be more than about 85 Cals / **357 kJ**.

20 yrs ago:
85 Cals
/ 357 kJ
Today:
Up to
480 Cals
/ 2016 kJ

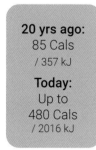
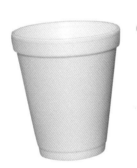
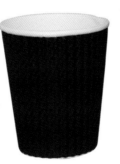
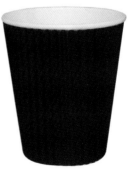
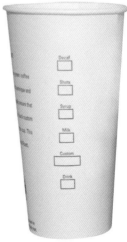

Over the last 15 or so years, though, there's been a coffee revolution. Where 20 years ago it wasn't that common to get a take-away – and many of us didn't even know what a latte was – now it's a different story. Think about the various different sizes of take-away cups, and all the milk-based coffees you can now order – lattes, flat whites and cappuccinos – and we start to see a problem. A regular milk-based coffee (and you can include hot chocolates here, too) would contain 200 Cals / 840kJ. That's a 'Regular' but what about a Grande? At 16.5 fl oz / 470 ml, a Grande provides up to 480 Cals / 2016 kJ, depending on the particular drink you've ordered.

Flavored milk

Twenty years ago, Flavored milk was sold in 10 fl oz / 300 ml cartons, containing 220 Cals / 924 kJ. Now 17- 21 fl oz / 500–600 ml is more the norm, and the Calorie count is up to 440 Cals / 1848 kJ. So a large milk drink doesn't go with lunch ... it IS lunch!

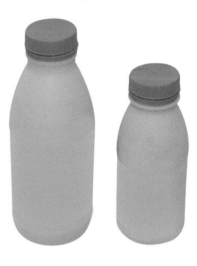

20 yrs ago:
220 Cals / 924 kJ
Today:
440 Cals / 1848 kJ

Crisps

Twenty years ago a small packet of crisps weighed 1 oz / 30 g, today both 1.8 oz / 50 g and 3.5 oz / 100 g packets are marketed as single servings.

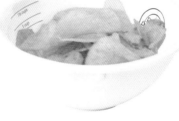

• **1 oz** / 30 g **= 150 Cals** / 630 kJ

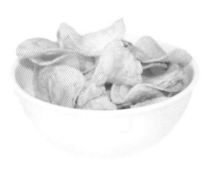

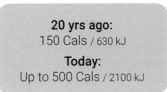

20 yrs ago:
150 Cals / 630 kJ
Today:
Up to 500 Cals / 2100 kJ

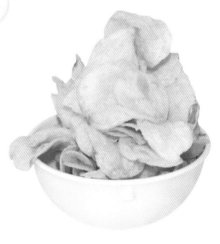

• **1.8 oz** / 50 g **= 250 Cals** / 1050 kJ

• **3.5 oz** / 100 g **= 500 Cals** / 2100 kJ

Cookies

Twenty years ago a choc chip cookie contained 50 Cals / 210 kJ. Today the jumbo cookies found in coffee shops can contain over 500 Cals / **2100 kJ**.

20 yrs ago: 50 Cals / 210 kJ
Today: 500 Cals / 2100 kJ

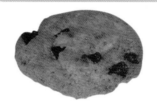
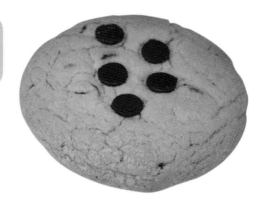

Sugary drinks

Now that manufacturers are pushing 21 fl oz / **600 ml** bottles of sugary drink as the 'normal' size, the smaller size is starting to look like a cute, old-fashioned model.

- A 16 fl oz / 450 ml bottle contains 180 Cals / 672 kJ – okay for an occasional snack if you're a healthy weight.

- A 21 fl oz / 600 ml bottle contains 245 Cals (1029 kJ) – a hefty addition to any meal.

You may not have thought of drinks as snacks before. Calorie-containing drinks are a significant contributor to energy overconsumption. Instead of thinking of it as 'just a drink', it's time to consider it as a food choice. If you're hungry choose something solid – not liquid.

20 yrs ago:
160 Cals / 672 kJ
Today:
245 Cals / 1029 kJ

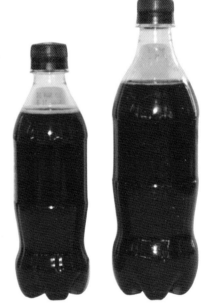

SLEEVE COMMENT: I cannot eat *AND* drink. I need about ¾ hour before and after meals. *Donna*

BAND COMMENT: Choosing solids, not liquids is a fundamental concept for lapband success given the tendency to seek liquid or softer options to avoid potential difficulties. *Cath*

BYPASS COMMENT: The reason I had surgery is to feel full and satisfied on a small amount of food and have that feeling of satiety stay with me as long as possible. Avoiding eating and drinking together helps me stay full longer. *Colleen*

Perfect Portions

So how did our portions get so big?

The main reason behind increasing portion size is simply that food manufacturers want to make more money, and they have a number of clever ways of achieving this.

Their aim is to persuade us to eat more of their products. There are two ways of doing this: they can sell more, although this isn't necessarily easy to do. The simpler option is to make the products bigger (and therefore more expensive).

Food is actually a fairly small component of the cost of a food product. The main costs are the labour, the packaging and the advertising. It is therefore a very cheap option to offer extra-large portions as an attractive offer to consumers. For example, you can get an upgrade on a take-away meal which gives you 50 per cent more food for 16 per cent more money. Or a company might decide to manufacture a 'king-sized' packet, which costs more, and then gradually phase out the original packaging size.

Another simple benefit of larger products from the manufacturer's point of view is: the bigger the packet, the more visible it is on the supermarket shelf. That huge packet of cornflakes acts like an advertising billboard in the supermarket.

Of course, consumers aren't entirely blameless, either. Where we fall down is that we are attracted to value for money deals – but is it value for money to eat more than you need? What is the actual cost in health and efforts to lose that excess weight gained? And don't forget the financial cost of surgery.

Value for money?

Our local donut franchise gives two free cinnamon donuts with every thickshake. For weight loss, the aim is 100 Calories for a snack. The thickshake itself is equivalent to a large meal at 530 Cals – add the donuts and you're up over 1000 Cals!

What we eat is certainly a problem for some, but *how much* we eat is becoming a problem for all of us.

Size Matters

Many food packets have recommended serving sizes on the nutrition information panel. These can be very misleading.

For example, look at the label for this divine-sounding dessert. The heading at the top of the nutrition information panel says 'per serve', 470 kJ, which is only just over 100 Cals. This sounds appealing, right? But think again. The pack weighs 7 oz / **200 g** – the same as a single-serve yogurt tub – so it would be easy to think it is a serve. It's only when you study the label that you find that there are five servings per pack. One serve equals roughly one spoonful!

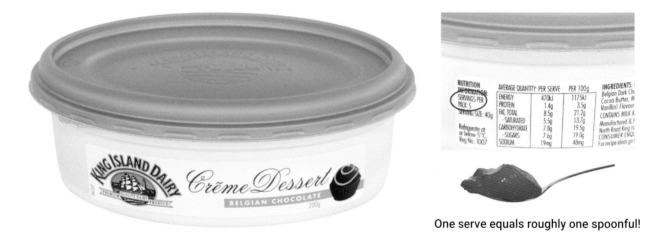

One serve equals roughly one spoonful!

Later in the book, I'll explain how to read labels to get the information you need. They might be misleading, but it's easy to find the information you need when you know what to look for. See page 48 for more details.

Although as I've explained, the portion sizes of packaged foods are out of control, there's no need for you to be bamboozled by them any longer. *Portion Perfection for Bariatrics* is here to make your life easier!

Chapter 2: The Portion Perfection Concept

There is much valuable research to show that the more food we put on our plates, the more we will eat. The scary thing is we often don't realize that we are eating more. When you have had bariatric surgery this can be a disaster for longterm success. Stomachs are stretchy membranes and the more times you stretch your stomach the more food it will hold before you sense satisfaction.

The research shows that the larger the plate the more we eat; the larger the spoon the more we eat, the larger the packet or serving bowl the more we eat, and the greater the variety on offer, the more we eat. All without significant awareness.

You may think you are too clever to be fooled by a larger bowl, but even nutrition experts get caught. One American study focused on 85 nutrition experts who were attending an ice cream celebration for a colleague. They were randomly given either a smaller (two cup) or larger (four cup capacity) bowl and either a 2 fl oz / 60 ml or 3 fl oz / 90 ml ice cream scoop. After serving themselves, their bowls were weighed while they completed a survey. This study found that the people who were given a larger bowl served themselves 31 per cent more without being aware of it. They even served an additional 14 per cent if they used the larger serving spoon. And these people were nutrition experts!

Portion Perfection Plates and Bowls work!

Apart from my own experience, others around the world are testing out the same theory. A review published in 2021 found that portion control plates lead to reductions in body weight, waist circumference, blood pressure and improved blood test results.

This is where the Portion Perfection concept comes in.

Introducing the tools

The Great Ideas in Nutrition Portion Perfection Bariatric Plates and Bowls serve as self-monitoring tools to help encourage healthy eating and weight loss.

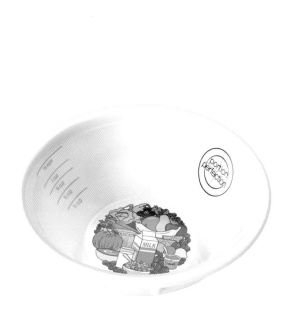

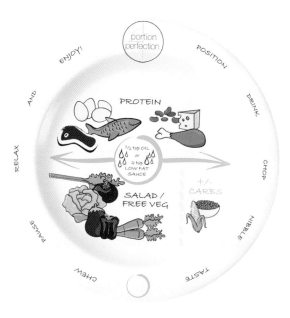

Portion Bowl - Melamine or Porcelain   Bariatric Plate - Melamine or Porcelain

The tools address three common issues:

1. Portion size
How much we eat depends largely on how much food we have on our plates or in the snack-food packet. Portion control is a valuable tool to add to your surgery.

2. Nutritional balance
Getting the right things for a balanced diet on your plate is easy with the plate system.

3. Eating awareness
By being fully aware of what you are eating, and eating in a 'conscious' way, you will find satisfaction for your mind as well as your stomach. This involves savouring your food and slowing down your eating so you feel satisfied with the smaller quantity. There are also specific eating behaviors that give you the best tolerance of foods after bariatric surgery. If you're open to the process of hypnotherapy, then our hypnotherapy audio can be a useful tool for keeping you on track.

Getting the right portion size

The Bariatric Plate is designed to hold approx 200–250 Cals / 840 - 1050kJ when the base is filled to a depth of ¾ inch / 2 cm, keeping the rim of the plate free of food. You should experience satisfaction on this amount if you have a recently formed sleeve or bypass or your band is adjusted correctly.

If you find that this amount of food is not enough to satisfy you, and you are a band owner, you may require an adjustment. When the plate is filled all the way to the edge, ¾ inch / 2 cm deep, it is approximately 350 Cals / 1470kJ which is a good limit to adhere to until your next band fill.

If you have had a sleeve or bypass and you are greater than 12 months post surgery, then you may have stretched your stomach pouch. Evidence suggests that by reducing your food intake as we show you here, you may not be able to shrink your stomach but you can calm the hunger messages such that you become comfortable on the smaller amount over about a week to 10 days.

The plates and bowls and hypnotherapy download are available from our website: www.portiondiet.com.

Finding the best nutritional balance for maximum healthy weight loss

The Portion Perfection Bariatric Plate is divided into segments which show the ideal proportion of protein foods to vegetables and carbohydrates for a balanced intake.

There is a small segment for carbohydrate foods which is essential if you have diabetes, but can otherwise be avoided at one meal per day to ensure Calorie intake is as low as practicable. Ideally, you should discuss how to best fill this segment with your dietitian.

If you are able to limit your carbohydrate intake at one meal per day, for example, dinner, then you leave ample space for protein foods and low-Calorie, nutrient-dense, high-fibre 'free vegetables'. This improves your overall nutritional intake.

We know that protein is more satisfying than either carbohydrate or fat, so protein is encouraged in the form of dairy or soy products, meat, fish, poultry, eggs or legumes. We've added protein counts like this **10** representing the number of grams of protein in that serve to help you ensure you're getting enough.

Satisfaction is the absence of hunger. Fullness means you've overstretched your stomach. Whenever you feel full, you've eaten too much.

SLEEVE COMMENT: If I overeat it is an uncomfortable feeling, like Christmas day when you know you have overdone it. Walking around seems to help the food go down. *Donna*

BAND COMMENT: For me, overeating or 'fullness' feels like pain, discomfort, distention, my port sticks out and I feel a risk of regurgitation. *Cath*

BYPASS COMMENT: Like most people, I do not like to be hungry. I don't like to be overfull either. I understand the importance of satiety and listen to my body's signals to help me know when to stop. As they say, one bite is the difference between being full and being sick. *Colleen*

The segments of the plate are to be filled by:

- Protein foods: lean red meat, poultry, fish, egg, legumes (soybeans, baked beans, lentils, chickpeas etc) or tofu.

- Low GI carbohydrates (This is specifically for those with diabetes. For others it may be nutritionally beneficial to omit this optional section in one main meal per day, eg. dinner): sweet potato/yams, peas, corn, basmati or doongara rice, pasta, rice noodles, grainy bread, a corn tortilla, couscous, quinoa, freekeh, bulgur, barley or spelt. This segment may also contain occasional amounts of baby potatoes, pita bread, parsnip, pumpkin, polenta or grits, which are all medium GI carbohydrates.

- Salads and free veg: alfalfa, artichoke, asparagus, bamboo shoots, bean sprouts, beets, broccoli, Brussels sprouts, cabbage, capsicum/peppers, eggplant/aubergine, green beans, leek, lemon, lettuce, marrow, mushrooms, onions, radish, rhubarb, rocket/arugula, shallots, silverbeet, snow peas, spinach, spring onion, squash, sugar snap peas, swede/rutabaga, tomato, turnip, water chestnut, watercress or zucchini/courgette.

- Sauces or dressings: oil or oily dressings, commercial low-fat dressings or those based on fruit juice or low-fat mayonnaise, skim milk sauces, low-fat gravy mixes, apple, honey-soy, oyster, mint, plum, BBQ, tomato, soy, hoisin, teriyaki, Worcestershire, chilli, sweet chilli, black bean or light (fat-reduced) cheese sauces.

Food Tolerance

Everyone is a little different when it comes to which foods are well tolerated. Band owner's tolerance is influenced by how tight the band is, the time of day, eating behaviour and individual factors. Our own research found that approximately 60% of band owners had difficulty tolerating white bread or red meat. Put another way, this means 1 in 3 had no problem with these foods. Don't assume that because others avoid certain foods, that you need to too. Sleeve recipients tend to experience less specific food tolerance problems and gastric bypass tends to cause some intolerance to starchy foods including rice, pasta and bread.

Easy meals to start with would be moist and low in starch like a stew, chilli or stir fry at dinner or a chicken or egg salad at lunch.

Another interesting outcome of our survey was that 100% of people who eat legumes such as baked beans, kidney beans, lentils and chickpeas experience no problems with these foods. To be sure of your own tolerance, follow the guidelines below for eating consciously.

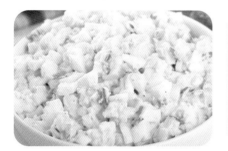 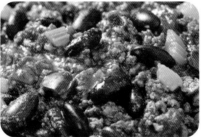 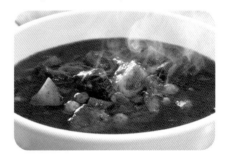

The Portion Perfection Bowl

The Portion Perfection Bowl is available from the website and indicates cup amounts. This is a useful adjunct to the plate and appears in the program photos in this book. The bowl can also be used for the puree phase to allow you to easily monitor food quantities. You can order via Amazon or www.portiondiet.com

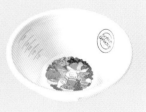

What is 'conscious eating'?

'Conscious eating' is a concept which comes from mindfulness psychology. It means eating with awareness, really looking at the food you intend to eat, smelling it, tasting it, savouring and enjoying it. This helps you reach satisfaction mentally as well as just filling the capacity of your stomach.

The words around the outside of the Portion Perfection Bariatric Plate prompt you to consider the following every time you eat.

How to eat consciously and get your eating behaviour right

Eating consciously is simple, but it may take some getting used to – you'll be surprised to find that it's something most people don't do! Slow down your eating and follow these steps for painless meals and snacks:

1. **Position** yourself to be sitting up straight. Slumping creates some upward pressure which can make it difficult for food to move smoothly into your small stomach.

2. **Drink** before your meal, When you have a band this can help to clear away any partially digested fibres left over from the previous meal. (These can result in regurgitation of frothy saliva.) Band owners can drink within minutes before a meal and have varying tolerance once they have started eating. Sleeve and Bypass owners need to allow more time before the meal to ensure the liquid has shifted out of the stomach. 30 – 45 minutes is recommended.

3. **Chop** your food well – check it against the circle on the plate border. It should be small enough to get through a space of that size. (This size is also the actual space available with a well adjusted gastric band, and will also apply to anyone with a band around their bypass or sleeve).

4. Take small bites (literally just **nibble**) to ensure that there is space for air to move up your oesophagus as food travels down. If you attempt to swallow too much food in one go, you may find it feels as though it is getting stuck part-way down. This is because there is air caught underneath the food which can't get past. In milder cases this can result in excessive burping.

5. Notice the **taste**, texture, temperature and aroma of the food.

6. **Chew** your food well. This is no substitute for chopping however. Often when we chew foods, we don't fully break the fibres – we just mash them up.

7. **Relax!** Tension creates upward pressure which can make it more difficult for food to go down.

8. Slow yourself right down and **enjoy!** Wait 90 seconds between mouthfuls.

To really get full enjoyment from eating, notice all the following attributes

- **Presentation** – before you start eating, notice the way the food looks. Has it been served in an attractive manner? Does it look appealing? Pay full attention to the quantity that you see – this will help you anticipate when the meal has ended. This is a good reason never to eat from a multi-serve packet – always serve out the amount you intend to eat, or buy single portion-sized packs.

- **Variety** – do you see a variety of colours, textures and types of foods on your plate?

- **Aroma** – smell the food. What do you notice? Does it smell fresh? Appetising? Can you smell all the components of the meal, or only some?

- As you eat the food, notice the **texture** – is it smooth? Grainy? Tough? Tender?

- Also think about the **temperature** – is it ideal for that particular food? Could it be warmer or cooler?

- Savour the **flavors** – what ingredients can you taste? Imagine if you didn't see what you put in your mouth. Do you think you could identify it from the taste and texture?

- And don't forget to slow yourself right down and **enjoy** the meal!

BAND COMMENT: These are critical points. *Cath*

SLEEVE COMMENT: These points work equally well for sleeve owners. *Donna*

BYPASS COMMENT: I love...the Portion Perfection bowl. What a "great idea!" it is important to take the guessing and wondering out of the equation and simply eat the right portions every time. *Colleen*

Liquid calories

With all bariatric surgeries, liquid calories will empty too quickly from the stomach and fail to produce relative satisfaction. The only time to choose liquid calories is when it is not convenient to eat solid food. For example, if you don't get a proper meal break, often a liquid such as milk or a protein shake may be tolerated by the workplace during the work day. Fruit based drinks are unlikely to be well tolerated by bypass patients due to risk of dumping.

CASE STUDIES

John

John leads a busy professional life as a lawyer. He consulted me for advice regarding having his gastric band removed. John had developed an embarrassing side effect, and was regurgiting frothy saliva regularly at business lunches. I explained to John the eating behaviours required to get the best tolerance with a gastric band, and he was able to understand the cause of the problem. He then factored in drinking 14 oz / 400 ml of water prior to attending lunch meetings, and chopping his food to appropriate sizes. Happily, his problems were solved without the need for further intervention.

Sonya

Sonya had spent most of her life feeling guilty about her eating habits and recognised that surgery might not change her attachments to certain foods. Our first discussion focused around conscious eating strategies. Sonya returned two weeks later, elated at the experience she'd had. She announced that she felt some freedom to enjoy foods and she even found that some of the foods she'd been clinging to for so long didn't taste that good. Sonya went on to have a sleeve gastrectomy to assist her to feel satisfied on a smaller volume of food, and consulted the clinic psychologist for coping strategies to replace food in her life.

Jane

Jane underwent Gastric Bypass five months ago and had lost an amazing 77 lb / 35 kg from her original 265 lb / 120 kg frame. She has developed a healthy interest in sport and is training for her first triathlon. Jane is fearful that she will be unable to achieve her nutritional and energy needs with her new smaller stomach, and might not be able to perform at her best. By showing Jane the everyday snacks with higher Calorie density, we were able to plan an ideal intake through the introduction of nuts and dried fruit. She was very pleased to complete her first triathlon and continues to train for further events.

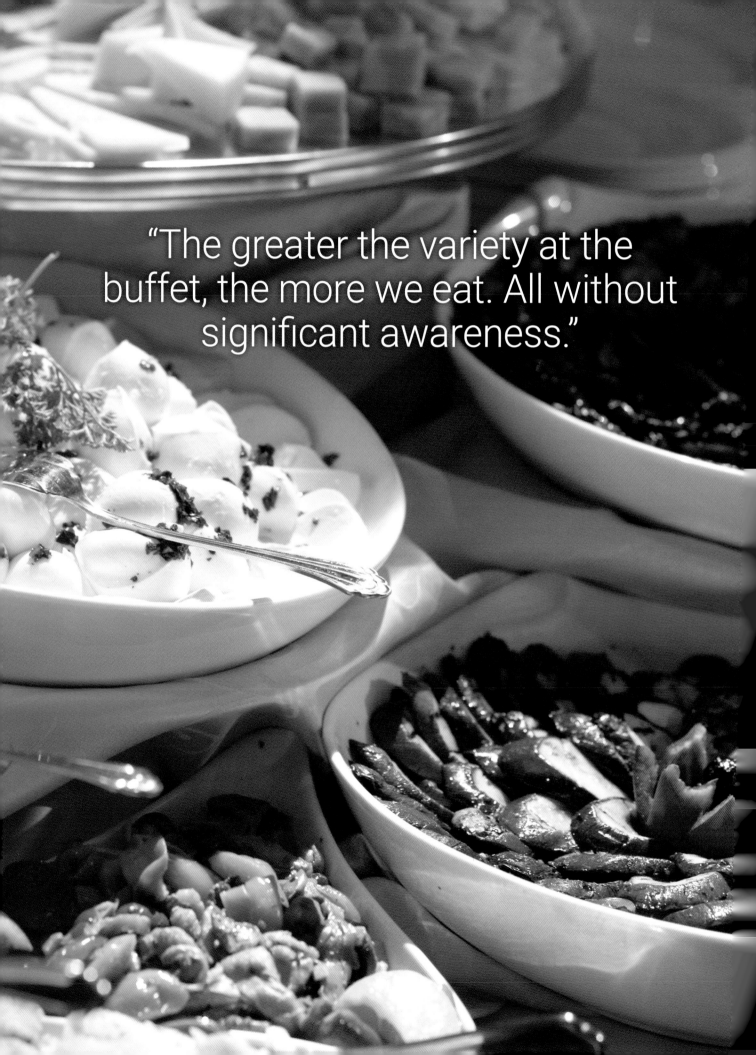

"The greater the variety at the buffet, the more we eat. All without significant awareness."

Chapter 3: Nutritional Considerations

There are several important nutritional considerations to be taken into account for those having undergone bariatric surgery. These are outlined in this chapter, together with general nutritional information to assist you in getting the most out of your Portion Perfection for Bariatrics kit.

Eating little and often

Most dieters report that the more diets they have been on, the harder it is to lose weight. When you think about it from an evolutionary point of view, it makes sense. Think of it this way: the more famines we live through, the more important it is for survival that our bodies become energy efficient – which means holding onto body fat as long as possible. This is a good reason to avoid cutting your Calorie intake too low without some expert advice.

How much should you cut your calorie intake by?

Not a lot of research has been done, however research does show that there is no benefit in reducing Calories below 800 / 3360 kJ per day. No additional body fat loss is achieved by eating 400 or 600 Cals / 1680-2520 kJ per day.

To snack or not to snack?

But what about how often to eat? Snacking is often discouraged by surgeons for fear of slowed weight loss. However, it's not necessary to cut out snacks entirely. Problems can be avoided by following this guide or your own dietitian's advice about smart and healthy snacking, so you still achieve your full weight loss potential.

One study on this area was carried out specifically on gastric band owners. It found that those who ate four or more meals per day lost more weight than those who ate three or less meals per day. To me that suggests snacks are important, but be guided by the recommendations of your team.

Aim for solid snack choices for best satisfaction.

Those who don't feel hungry between meals or who have difficulty getting those snacks in during work may benefit from a milk drink rather than skipping the snack altogether.

Nutritional needs for the 3 main forms of surgery differ slightly and this is explained below.

Sleeve Gastrectomy

Sleeve owners are specifically at risk of Vitamin B12 deficiency. A factor known as "Intrinsic Factor" is essential for the absorption of Vitamin B12 further down the digestive tract. Less stomach lining means less Intrinsic Factor is produced. A deficiency can develop over time. Generally a specific bariatric multivitamin along with Vitamin B12 and Vit D supplements are recommended.

Gastric Bypass

Because a portion of your small intestine has been bypassed, some nutrients will not be well absorbed from your food. Most surgeons require their patients take a bariatric multivitamin daily, and add to this a specific calcium supplement along with Vit D, B12 and iron supplements.

Your dietitian may recommend other supplements based on individual need. If you do not have access to a dietitian and would like a nutritional analysis completed, please contact me via our website.

Gastric Banding

Because the digestive system is virtually unchanged, this form of surgery has the least specific nutritional problems. The main problem is that your food volume drops below that critical 8 cup level required to ensure nutritional intake. For this reason a multivitamin is recommended. Nutrients commonly found to be consumed in low amounts by gastric band owners include folic acid, calcium, iron, B12 and thiamine. A chewable version is best tolerated. Additional Vit D and calcium may also be recommended depending on intake and blood results.

Research shows a high incidence of malnutrition in people undergoing weight loss surgeries. It is important that your nutritional status be assessed prior to surgery as poor nutritional status can lead to suboptimal immunity and wound healing, which places you at risk of infection. Ongoing yearly reviews by your health team are also recommended. Persisting deficiencies will lead to problems such as anaemia and osteoporosis if not addressed.

Developing a meal plan structure can help to ensure you cover your needs. The following meal plan combines perfectly with the recommended vitamin supplements to cover all your nutritional needs. Note the recommendations for your surgery but be guided by your dietitian.

- **Breakfast:** cereal, milk and fruit, bariatric multivitamin
- **AM snack:** fruit
- **Lunch:** wholegrain crackers with meat and salad, iron supplement (bypass)
- **PM snack:** dairy-based snack, calcium supplement (all or as advised)
- **Dinner:** meat/chicken/fish and free vegetables, and second bariatric multivitamin (all)
- **Supper snack:** dairy-based snack, second calcium supplement (all or as advised).

When you reach your goal weight, you may be able to start increasing your calorie intake. Consult with your dietitian about whether switching to the standard version of Portion Perfection, starting on the lower calorie level and gradually building up until your weight is stable.

At goal weight, there will be room for the less nutrient – dense everyday options like some of the healthier muesli bars. This will make it easier to reach your optimum nutritional intake and leave space for some less healthy 'occasional' options. So there is a light at the end of the tunnel.

BAND COMMENT: I found this weight loss phase liberating, not punishing. It was strange and unfamiliar rather than difficult. *Cath*

SLEEVE COMMENT: I had always eaten healthy and I found the restrictive amount of food is great. I don't get hypos anymore and am free of the urge to overeat. *Donna*

BYPASS COMMENT: Throughout my nearly 20 years as a bypass patient, I have adopted many new habits. When it comes to my food choices I am always mindful to eat enough protein each day, avoid sugary foods and drinks and be careful with breads, grains, pasta, crackers etc. *Colleen*

Carbohydrates

You'll notice that carbohydrates feature in most meals – this is because they are the best fuel for your muscles and brain. It is okay to omit them in one main meal per day to leave extra space for protein and low starch vegetables or salad. Talk to your dietitian about the best option for you.

A word on carbohydrates

It's important not to be fooled into thinking we weren't designed to eat them; that's what the enzymes in our intestines are for. Over half the world's population lives on carbohydrate-based foods as their staple – and most of those people don't have the obesity problem that we do in the Western world, so that is not the answer. It's just that carbohydrates aren't essential for every meal.

Protein

Protein is vital for maintaining muscle mass and therefore metabolic rate as you lose weight. Protein is also essential to the structure of red blood cells, the immune system, the regulation of enzymes and hormones and for healing after surgery.

Daily protein needs will be calculated by your dietitian and for most people this will be in the range of 60-90g protein per day and may depend on your type of surgery. I recommend using a protein supplement daily to provide 20 - 30g of protein. This takes the pressure off all the food you eat having to be high protein, leaving space for nutritious vegetables, fruits and grains.

To help you ensure that you are achieving your daily intake we have displayed the protein content of each choice. For example, ½ cup cottage cheese, shown on page 59 contains **13** grams of protein and is a very good choice because it may provide one third of daily needs.

Drinks

Timing your intake of liquids is important to get the best from your bariatric procedure. I recommend drinking before meals. With a band, thin liquids such as water can be consumed within minutes before starting a meal because they will simply slide through in to the second pouch. You may also find that you can drink small sips approximately 2 minutes after a mouthful of food, though experiences vary. With a sleeve or bypass, you may be able to drink water on an empty stomach within about 10 minutes before a meal. Water will pass out of your stomach fairly quickly because there is nothing to be digested. After a meal, however, a 30 - 40 minute delay is required to ensure the stomach space has cleared of food and there is sufficient space for fluid.

The type of liquid you drink is also important. Liquids will generally not be as satisfying as solid food. Keep most of your Calories for solid food, and limit Calories from drinks to 7 fl oz / 200 ml milk. A milk drink can be handy if you don't get the opportunity to eat a solid snack between meals. Check out the volume of your glasses – use large glasses for water and small 7 fl oz / 200 ml glasses for milk.

Making sense of milks

Once upon a time, milk was milk, but now it comes in many forms. It can be confusing to know what is best for you.

Originally, alternatives to cow's milk were the choice of those experiencing intolerance or allergy to cow's milk, whilst now the reasons for choosing alternatives are many and varied.

Nutritionally, milks vary significantly. The following comparison shows that cow's milk is unbeatable for protein, but almond milk is a very low Calorie alternative. Carbohydrate content is lowest in almond milk and highest in rice milk. Calcium does not occur naturally in significant quantities in almonds, soy beans, rice or coconut so check the label on your brand of these milks to note how the fortification level compares to cow's milk's natural levels. Throughout this book, choose quantities of milk based on the final column of number of mls for 100 Cals. That is, in the snack section, where 100 Cals of milk is included, use 150ml full cream dairy milk or 600ml almond milk or 300ml rice milk.

Milk	Cals per cup (200 ml)	Carbs (g)	Sugars (g)	Fat (g)	Sat Fat (g)	Protein (g)	100 Cal serve (ml)	50 Cal 'mini' serve (ml)
Full cream dairy	160 Cals / 672 kJ	11	11	8	5	8	150	75
Low fat dairy (1%)	110 Cals / 462 kJ	12	12	2.5	1	8	200	100
Fat Free dairy (0%)	90 Cals / 378 kJ	13	12	0	0	8	250	125
Almond	30 Cals / 126 kJ	1	0	3	<1	1	600	300
Coconut	45 Cals / 189 kJ	2	0	4	4	0	400	200
Hemp	140 Cals / 588 kJ	19	12	6	1	4	200	100
Oat	107 Cals / 446 kJ	21	13	4	1	2	200	100
Rice	140 Cals / 588 kJ	30	14	2.5	0	0	300	150
Soy	110 Cals / 462 kJ	9	6	4.5	0.5	8	200	100

Reference: Walmart online common brands 2022. Look for protein increased versions.

Cow's Milk is widely available and comes in varying modified forms including reduced fat, fat free, lactose free and A2. Some people choose to avoid cow's milk due to intolerance or ethical concerns. Full fat cow's milk contains significant levels of saturated fats.

Almond Milk is made from ground almonds and filtered water. There may also be added starches or thickeners and it comes in sweetened and unsweetened varieties. Those who are allergic to nuts should avoid almond milk. Almond milk contains no saturated fat, but does contain healthy unsaturated fats. It is low in calories, and almond milk may be fortified with calcium. It is not naturally a good source of protein but some protein increased products are available.

Coconut Milk is made from grated and filtered coconut flesh and water. The drinking version is more dilute than the coconut milk used for cooking. Coconut milk may contain added thickeners. The fat in coconut milk is saturated. Coconut milk is not generally associated with allergic reactions and contains a component of medium chain triglycerides (MCT) which may hold some benefit for weight control. Coconut milk is not a good source of protein, and check the label for calcium fortification.

Hemp Milk is made from ground hemp seeds and filtered water. Hemp seeds or milk do not contain any of the psychoactive component of marijuana. Hemp milk has a nutty flavor and is high in unsaturated fats including plant based omega 3 fatty acids. Hemp milk may contain added sugars and may be fortified with calcium.

Oat milk is made from whole oats or oat flour, blended with filtered water and oil. There may be added sugar. Oat milk is free of saturated fat, may be fortified with calcium and is naturally low to moderate in protein but protein increased products are available. An added benefit is the presence of beta glucan – known to assist with cholesterol control. Oat milk is also the highest fibre milk, containing up to 2 g per glass.

Rice Milk is made from ground rice and filtered water. It is naturally sweet and may contain thickeners. Rice has high tolerance due to low protein content. It may be fortified with calcium. Some concerns regarding arsenic content have spiked warnings in the US to limit rice milk in children.

Soy Milk is made from ground soy beans and filtered water but may also contain sugars and starches for flavor and texture. Soy milk is a good source of protein and may be fortified with calcium. Some people choose to avoid soy milk for reasons of intolerance, health or agricultural concerns.

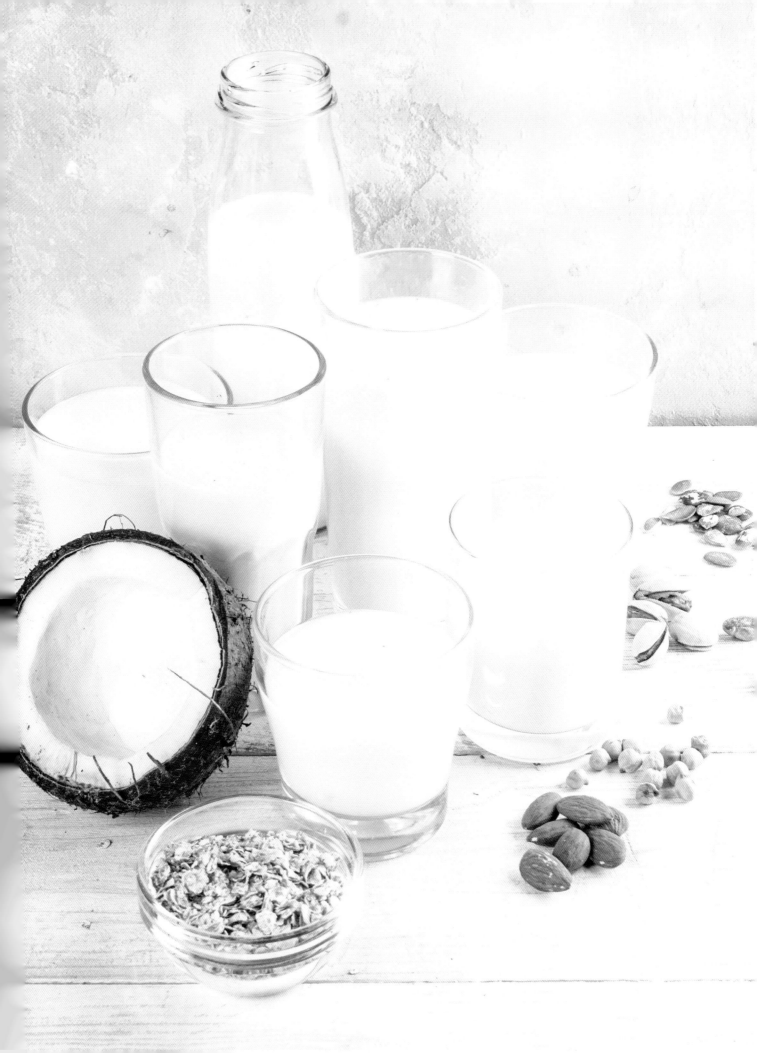

The Glycemic Index

The Glycemic Index (GI) is a rating system for food, showing you how quickly each type of food raises your blood sugar levels. Foods with a high GI raise blood sugar levels quickly while low GI foods produce a more gradual rise. For example, sweet potato/yam gives a slow rise, whereas common forms of potato produce a quick rise in blood sugar. The benefits of a lower GI diet include feeling more satisfied, a more stable mood, fewer cravings for sweet or starchy foods and better energy levels. Low GI foods also lower your insulin levels, which can help to burn stored fat. All positive things to help you avoid the seemingly inevitable weight creep!

The chart below provides some GI basics and explains why some seemingly healthy foods have ended up in the occasional category.

	HIGH GI FOODS	LOWER GI ALTERNATIVES
Breads	Whole wheat and white breads	Bread high in whole grains or low in carbohydrates
Cereals	Processed, low fibre and sugary breakfast cereals	Higher fibre, lower sugar cereals and those based on traditional or steel cut oats
Cookies/Crackers	Plain cookies and crackers, rice-based crackers and bars	Cookies made with dried fruit or whole grains such as oats
Cakes	Cakes and muffins	Look for those made with fruit, oats or whole grains
Fruit	Cantaloupe, watermelon, lychees	Temperate climate fruits such as apples and stone fruit, pears and oranges, greenish bananas, berries, kiwi fruit, mango, or pawpaw
Starchy vegetables, legumes and pasta	Most common forms of potato	Pasta, legumes (baked beans, lentils etc), sweet potato/yam, Carisma potato, peas or corn
Rice	Most white rices, especially jasmine	Basmati or Doongara rice or medium grain brown rice
Dairy	Sorbet	Skim or low-fat milk (plain or flavored), yogurt, custard, low-fat ice cream and dairy desserts

Everyday, Vital and Occasional foods

In the Food Guide section of the book, which starts on page 57, foods have been divided into the following categories:

Everyday foods are low G.I., low in fat and provide moderate to high levels of valuable nutrients.

Vital is a category introduced in the snack section which denotes the snack foods which are high in critical nutrients. Choose these snacks 90% of the time.

Occasional meals may be higher in fat or lower in nutritional value and are best kept to an intake of twice per week or less. Occasional snacks in this book are actually still pretty healthy. They do however contain lower levels of critical nutrients and are best included in the 'twice a week' category.

During the weight loss phase following surgery, choose an occasional meal or snack no more than twice per week. Choosing healthier foods will boost your energy levels.

Diabetes

What if you have diabetes? Well, the good news is that this book will work for you, too. Nutrition guidelines for Type 2 diabetes or pre-diabetes (impaired glucose tolerance) set out by Diabetes organisations around the world indicate that meals should be:

1. Regular and spread evenly throughout the day

2. Low in fat, particularly saturated fat

3. Based on low GI carbohydrate foods such as wholegrain breads, cereal, lentils, vegetables and fruit.

Along with healthy eating, regular physical activity can help to manage and maintain a healthy weight.

These are the same principles applied in this book, so you can be confident that following the *Portion Perfection for Bariatrics* guide will contribute to positive outcomes in diabetes prevention and control. For further assistance, or if you are taking insulin or medication for either Type 2 or Type 1 diabetes, consult your Registered Dietitian.

Consider an indulgent dose of 'occasional' foods like a trip to Tahiti. Most of us can't afford to go very often, but as long as we know we can go occasionally, we don't feel too deprived!

"...the bigger the serving spoon,
the more we eat."

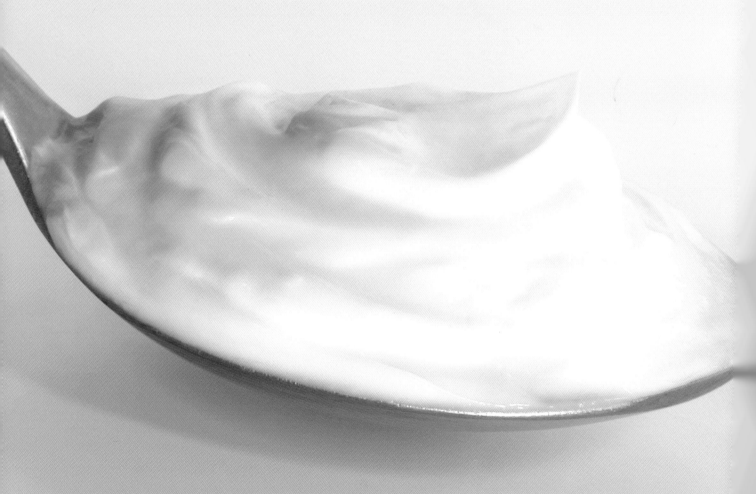

Chapter 4: Portion Perfection in Practice

Your surgeon will have set a goal weight for you at the time of surgery. See the BMI chart below as a guide. Knowing where you're headed and how to interpret food labels to ensure you get there – and stay there – are imperative.

To result in weight loss you need to consume fewer Calories than you are burning off. Most of us tend not to do exactly the same amount of activity every day, but as long as the intake is less than the expenditure, then weight loss should result. Some of us will lose weight faster than others, and some slower, depending on height, starting weight, muscle mass and exercise. In short, weight loss is an inexact science!

Maintaining weight is perhaps a bit more exact – to maintain, you need roughly equal energy intake and output. Depending on whether you reached a weight plateau on the *Portion Perfection for Bariatrics* meal plan, it may be appropriate for you to increase your calorie intake for maintenance. For example, when John (see the case study on page 33) reached his goal weight he started on 1600 Cals / 6720kJ then moved to an intake of 2200 Calories / 9240kJ, however he regained 4.5 lb / 2 kg slowly. We then reduced the size of his snacks which resulted in weight maintenance.

If you have specific needs or metabolic problems, I'd encourage you to consult a bariatric nutrition professional who will be able to review your profile and personalise your plan. In the US go to www.eatright.org and click on Find a Registered Dietitian. In the UK go to www.freelancedietitians.org. In Australia go to www.anzmoss.com.au and click on the Nutrition tab.

Dietitians recommend an acceptable rate of weight loss to be anything between 2 pounds / 1kg per week and 2 pounds / 1kg per month for adults and teenagers over 13. Faster weight loss may occur in the initial stages after surgery. This is fine because while your bariatric procedure is working for you there is minimal risk of weight regain with the right eating habits.

'Weight regain is a risk with all bariatric operations. Most patients will lose weight initially; however, the key to long-term success is developing good eating habits and making permanent lifestyle changes. Falling back into old habits will counteract the effects of the surgery'.

Mr Krishna Epari, Bariatric Surgeon

What weight is right for me?

A simple way to assess your ideal weight is by using the Body Mass Index (BMI). This is a general measure of body mass, and provides a good general guide to whether you are underweight, average, or overweight. Higher BMIs result in higher risk for diabetes, heart disease and joint problems.

Calculate your BMI using one of the following equations:

Your weight (pounds) ÷ your height (inches)^2 and multiply this answer by 703 = your BMI

OR Your weight (kg) ÷ your height (m)^2 = your BMI

BMI 18.5–25 = Healthy weight

BMI 25–30 = Moderate health risk

BMI 30+ = High to very high health risk

Note: The BMI is useful as a general guide, however it does not take individual muscle mass into consideration. Many people who have reached a very high body weight have also achieved a very high muscle mass. It is beneficial to maintain as much of that muscle mass as possible, as muscle determines how many Calories your body burns. For a true assessment of your ideal weight, consult a dietitian with access to body composition equipment.

Weight Regain

Whilst bariatric surgery is the most effective weapon against obesity, weight regain still occurs. It may start around 2 years after surgery and continue for several years before finding a new settling point. This occurs for many reasons and may reach 15 - 25% of weight lost. Common reasons for weight regain include our bodies working their way around the changes of surgery, introduction of grazing behaviour, increasing portion sizes or return to other habits that may have led to the original weight gain. I recommend maintaining contact with your team beyond the first year after surgery as accountability is a strong motivator. If you don't have a team and would like additional support please contact us.

How much do I need?

The daily Calorie guide that this book is based on is as follows:

Breakfast: 200–250 Cals (840–1050 kJ), and up to 1 cup	**Morning snack:** 100 Cals (420 kJ) and up to 1 cup
Lunch: 200–250 Cals (840–1050 kJ) and up to 1 cup	**Afternoon snack:** 100 Cals (420 kJ) and up to 1 cup
Dinner: 200–250 Cals (840–1050 kJ) and up to 1 cup	**Supper:** 100 Cals (420 kJ) and up to 1 cup

Everyone is a little different when it comes to hunger sensation and the amount your stomach stretches, so if you find that you are not achieving a weight loss of between 0.5 lb / 0.25kg and 4.5 lb / 2 kg per week, you should consult a bariatric dietitian who will modify the plan. For example, they may recommend that you eat 350 Cals / 1470 kJ per meal by adding the snack to mealtimes.

Remember that lowering Calories below 1100 Cals / 4620 kJ per day is only beneficial to those who have undergone weight loss surgery and that there is no benefit at all from lowering Calories below 800 Cals / 3360 kJ.

How to read food labels

Nutrition information labeling requirements vary between countries but the things that mislead us are universal. It is difficult to suggest the right nutritional content per serve because each company determines their own serving size and often it doesn't relate to a size that we would perceive to be one serve.

Where a "per 100g" set of data is provided, use this to compare between products to choose the better one.

Use the per serve figures to decide whether the number of Calories in the serve are right for your needs and check whether their statement of a serve size is realistic.

The produce labels shown are in Australian, US and UK formats for the same product. Note for each of them that the container holds 5 serves.

Decide whether this food is a meal or a snack and check your Calorie target and remember the goal of 200 – 250 Cals / 840 - 1050 kJ for meals and 100 Cals / 420 kJ for snacks.

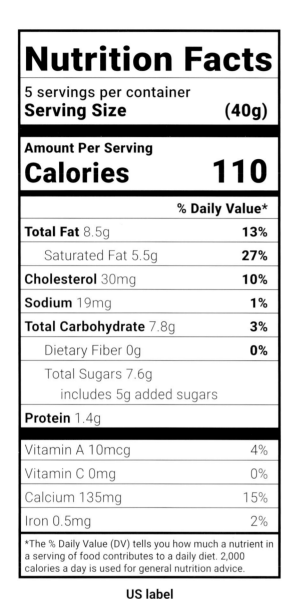

Nutrition Facts

5 servings per container
Serving Size (40g)

Amount Per Serving
Calories 110

	% Daily Value*
Total Fat 8.5g	**13%**
Saturated Fat 5.5g	**27%**
Cholesterol 30mg	**10%**
Sodium 19mg	**1%**
Total Carbohydrate 7.8g	**3%**
Dietary Fiber 0g	**0%**
Total Sugars 7.6g	
includes 5g added sugars	
Protein 1.4g	
Vitamin A 10mcg	4%
Vitamin C 0mg	0%
Calcium 135mg	15%
Iron 0.5mg	2%

*The % Daily Value (DV) tells you how much a nutrient in a serving of food contributes to a daily diet. 2,000 calories a day is used for general nutrition advice.

US label

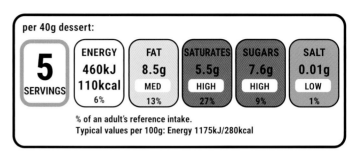

per 40g dessert:

5 SERVINGS	ENERGY 460kJ 110kcal 6%	FAT 8.5g MED 13%	SATURATES 5.5g HIGH 27%	SUGARS 7.6g HIGH 9%	SALT 0.01g LOW 1%

% of an adult's reference intake.
Typical values per 100g: Energy 1175kJ/280kcal

UK label

Nutrition Information:

Servings Per Package: 5
Serving Size (40g)

	Avg. Quantity per serving	Avg. Quantity per 100g
Energy	460kJ	1175kJ
Protein	1.4g	3.5g
Fat Total	8.5g	21.2g
– Saturated Fat	5.5g	13.7g
Carbohydrate	7.8g	19.5g
– Sugars	7.6g	19.0g
Sodium	19mg	48mg

Australian label

What else is on the label?

You'll also find on the label information about:

- **Protein**: Protein helps you feel more satisfied and keeps your blood sugar levels steady. Your daily requirement is likely to be 60–90 g. This figure will give you a feel for whether the product is a good source of protein or not. The pictured product is fairly low in protein, at 1.4 g per serve.

- **Fat**: This is often broken down into total fat and saturated fat, while some products may also list unsaturated fats and omega 3 fatty acids. In general you want no more than one-third of the fat in the food to be saturated. A low-fat food generally contains less than 10 g of fat if it is a meal in itself or less than 5 g of fat if it is a snack. The pictured product is a little high in fat for an everyday snack, and the fat is primarily saturated. This product is better substituted by a vital dairy snack during the weight loss phase.

- **Carbohydrate**: This is broken down into total carbohydrate and sugars. One trick is that the 'sugars' figure includes naturally occurring sugars in any fruit in the product as well as any milk ingredient. You will need to look at the ingredient list to get a feel for where the sugar is coming from. In general look for less than 5 g of added sugar for a snack or less than 10 g for a meal. Higher sugar intakes can be acceptable if there is more than 2 g of fibre in the snack or if it is based on fruit. The carbohydrate reading is not a good indicator of the Glycemic Index of a food.

The pictured product opposite, contains 7.8 g of carbohydrate, of which 7.6 g is sugar. This is a milk-based product so we know some of that sugar is actually the lactose in the milk. If you refer back to the GI chart on page 42, you will see that most dairy products are low GI even when they have added sugar. The sugar is therefore absorbed fairly slowly, making this a 'better' source of sugar.

- **Fibre**: High fibre foods generally have higher nutritional value and lower GI. Look for products with more than 3 g of fibre per 100 g, or more than 8 g per 100 g for breakfast cereals. The pictured product does not contain a fibre listing, and, being a milk product, would not be expected to contain significant fibre.

- **Sodium**: This is important for those on a sodium-restricted diet. Foods are considered to be low salt if they contain less than 120 mg of sodium per 100 g of food. Moderate salt foods usually contain less than 450 mg per 100 g of product. The pictured product would qualify as a low salt food.

There may be other nutritional components shown on the labels that you read; however, those listed above are the important ones for our purpose.

The ingredients on any packet are listed in order from the largest to the smallest amount based on weight of the ingredient. This will give you an indication of how naturally nutritious the product really is. Look for real food ingredients like fruit, milk, grains etc. You will be surprised at the number of chemical names on some food product labels. The ingredients list for this product includes Pasteurised Cream, Skim Milk, Belgian Dark Chocolate, Cocoa Butter, Milk Solids, Emulsifiers, Flavor and Vegetable Gums. Cream being the first ingredient on the list explains this products high saturated fat content. The chemical content is quite low and most of the additives listed (vegetable gums and emulsifiers) are not commonly associated with any adverse reactions.

This product could be classified as an occasional food, and a 100 Calorie / 420 kJ snack would be approximately one spoonful. This amount would not make a satisfying snack even after bariatric surgery. This product would not be recommended as a snack until maintenance is achieved and calorie intake increases.

Supplements

Research shows that a significant proportion of patients undergoing weight loss surgery have poor eating habits which means that they will be at further risk after surgery of suboptimal wound healing and decreased resistance to infection. Most surgeons now use dietary principles and a dietitian to prepare their patients for surgery. This often incudes two to four weeks of a low calorie, low carbohydrate, high nutrient quality diet.

After surgery, when intake is restricted to small volumes, the quality of each mouthful becomes critical. It is for this reason that bariatric multivitamin and mineral supplements are generally recommended.

Below is a sample of a healthy intake for anyone having undergone bariatric surgery and having passed the initial post surgery phases. This should be combined with the recommended supplementation regime as per page 37. Note delays between fluids and foods are as per page 38.

Breakfast: 10.5 oz / 300 ml reduced fat smoothie with 1 scoop protein powder 20

Morning snack: Slice of cheese 5

Lunch: 3 oz / 90 g tandoori chicken breast accompanied by ½ cup of green salad with dressing 22

Afternoon snack: Coffee, then 1 cup of canned fruit 1

Dinner: 3.3 oz / 100 g fish plus broccoli and carrots 28

Supper: 5 oz / 150 g Yogurt 11

Total protein = 87 g

Bariatric procedures do nothing magical to make body fat disappear. That's where you come in.

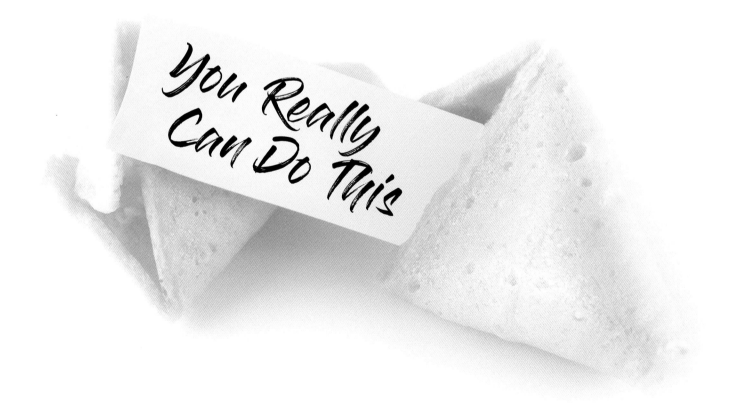

A nutritional analysis shows that this intake does not meet all your nutritional needs. The bars in purple in the graph below represent the percentage of the recommended dietary intake achieved through diet alone. The green bars show the change achieved with the addition of a bariatric specific multivitamin.

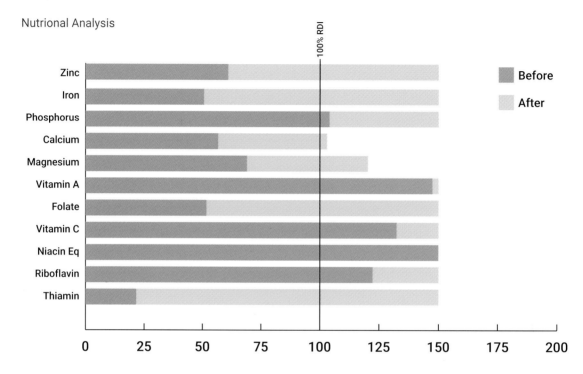

% Recommended Dietary Intake

(Please note it is not necessarily better to achieve intakes significantly higher than 100%.)

Making it work

To help achieve your goal of weight loss, in addition to following the guides shown in this book, you could:

1. Use the Portion Perfection for Bariatrics plate and bowl routinely and check for other Portion Perfection products helpful to you. The Bari-Kit-n-karry lunch bag is perfect for taking meals and snacks out with you. Enjoy using the Perfection wine glasses, pack leftovers from the *4 Week Weight Loss Menu Plan* recipe book into the Bari-preppers and carry snacks in the Portion Perfection Snacker. We've got you covered!

2. Work out the ideal quantities of your favourite foods and enter them in the notes section on each meal's title page within this book. I recommend Allan Borushek's *Calorie, Fat and Carbohydrate Counter* and the *Calorieking* smartphone app to help with this exercise in the US and Australia, and *My Fitness Pal* in the UK.

3. Keep a food diary - written or electronic.

4. Break leftovers down into appropriate portions. Ensure you package and refrigerate or freeze leftovers as soon as you have served your meal to avoid going back for seconds.

5. Buy smaller packages, focusing on those that contain a single serve per pack – or portion out larger packages to save cost and packaging.

6. Check in with your dietitian annually to check the adequacy of your intake and review your goals.

7. Develop a healthy attitude to portion control. Feel that you have ultimate flexibility vs restriction. Try reading Dr Rick Kausman's book *If Not Dieting Then What?* Change needs to be permanent. Dr George Blair West's book, *Weight Loss for Food Lovers, Understanding the Psychology and Sabotage of Weight Loss*, presents another useful approach.

8. Listen to the Portion Perfection Hypnotherapy MP3 daily.

9. Do regular resistance training. Resistance bands are a useful tool for building strength at home.

Try to include some incidental activity such as walking to get the paper or using the stairs instead of the lift, so that exercise isn't a chore.

Naturally exercise choice needs to be appropriate for your stage in the weight loss process and any physical limitations. In general I recommend minimum 30 minutes of aerobic activity daily to start with. However, it should be noted that to lose weight or maintain weight loss, 60 to 90 minutes of physical activity may be necessary. I also recommend muscle-toning exercise to maintain or increase strength and metabolic rate.

For more information on setting up a healthy exercise program, consult a physical therapist, qualified trainer or speak to your doctor.

Chapter 5: Food Guide Basics

Welcome to the food guide. This section is divided into meals, starting with breakfast, and moving on through lunch and dinner followed by a section on snacks, which are morning snack, afternoon snack and supper.

Generic products are shown that meet recommended criteria and come in the right portion size so you can easily find the best choices.

The plan represented here is designed to provide 800–1050 Cals / 3360–4410 kJ and all nutritional needs with the addition of the recommended supplements (see Chapter 4). The meals contain 200 - 250 Cals / 840 - 950 kJ and the snacks contain 100 Cals / 420 kJ. The protein content of each food or meal is shown e.g. **3** (grams). See page 38 to determine your needs. We recommend occasionally adding up your daily total to ensure you meet your needs.

Instructions:

1. Move to the appropriate section of the Food Guide for the meal of choice, for example, breakfast on page 57.

2. Select a menu option (note the recommended limits on occasional choices), and turn to that page.

3. Note the appropriate portion serve and prepare your meal accordingly.

Everyday choices have a green border on the page and occasional choices have a purple border.

Note the hints and tips for recipe selection. Our 4 Week Weight Loss Menu Plan is the perfect solution or choose your own favorite healthy cookbooks. Additional resources can be found in the Appendix at the back of this book. You don't need a special bariatric surgery cookbook – you really can eat most foods if you follow the guidelines around the outside of your plate.

Now you're ready to perfect your portions! Enjoy!

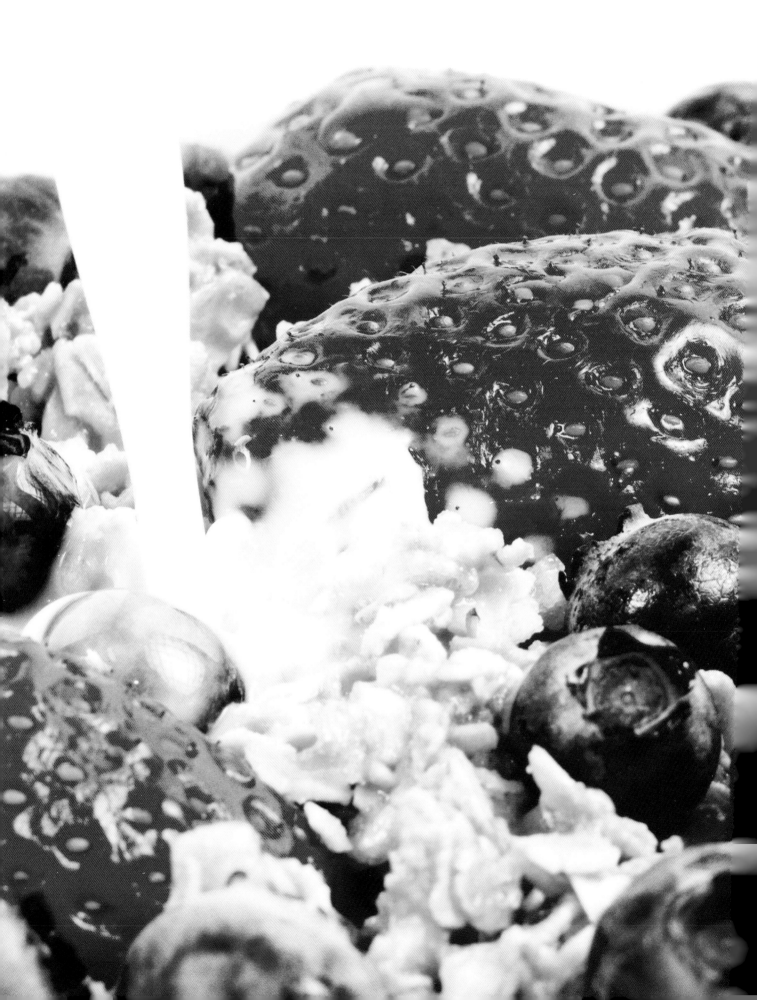

breakfast

This is the most socially acceptable time to eat fibre, so you don't want to miss the opportunity. The highest fibre choice is a bran-based cereal or baked beans. Many band owners experience poorer food tolerance in the morning. This is likely to be due to a redistribution of fluid after lying down all night. The tissues of the stomach lining are plumper, making the aperture for food to pass through smaller. As the day goes on, fluid gradually drains to the lower extremities by gravity, opening the aperture.

Breakfast kick starts the metabolism and there is clear evidence that concentration levels are improved in the morning following breakfast. We also know what those who skip breakfast end up eating more Calories than those who eat first thing in the morning.

For those who have trouble eating solid food of a morning, choose pureed fruit and yogurt or a smoothie for the best start to the day.

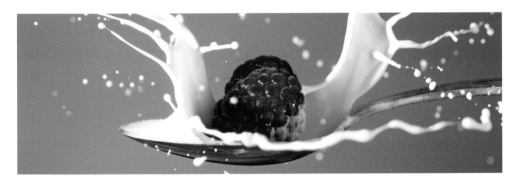

menu   page

Toast and topping 58
Cereal, fruit and milk 60
Yogurt and fruit 64
Smoothie 66
Omelette 67
Legumes 68

Add your own favourites by calculating a 200 Cal / 840 kJ serve via *Calorieking* in the US or Australia or *My Fitness Pal* in the UK.

Breakfast

Toast and toppings

Toast can be a great way to start the day, but is it too much to have melted cheese on it? Consider the components of a toast-based breakfast to be the bread, nutritious toppings to accompany the toast (Add Ons) and other choices that don't significantly add to the Calories but enhance the meal (free foods).

Meal components

Calories	Breads (100 Cals / 420 kJ)	Add Ons (100 Cals / 420 kJ)	Free Foods (<20 Cals / 85 kJ)
220 Cals / 924 kJ	1	1	1

Toast (100 Cals / 420 kJ)

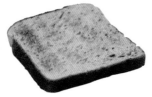

Wholegrain bread, 1 slice, 1 oz / 30 g **3**

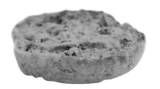

English muffin, ½, wholegrain **4** or fruit **3**

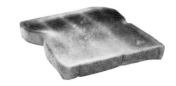

Low GI white bread, 1 slice, 1 oz / 30 g **3**

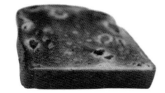

Raisin bread, 1 slice, 1 oz / 30 g **3**

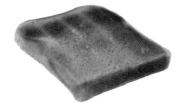

Stoneground whole wheat or sourdough rye, 1 slice, 1 oz / 30 g **3**

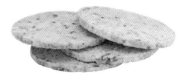

Grainy corn/rice cakes, 4 **3**

 Ensure toast is crisp – not soggy or doughy; sometimes stale is best.

"Breakfast kickstarts the metabolism and there is clear evidence that concentration levels are improved in the mornings following breakfast."

3 = Protein in grams.

Breakfast

Toast and toppings *continued*

Add Ons (100 Cals / 420 kJ)

* For more 'Add Ons' serves refer to Appendix 2

Note you may choose to have half of two Add Ons for your 100 Cals, rather than one whole Add On.
For example you might like the 1½ tsp spread with half a banana.

Cottage cheese, low fat,
½ cup / 4 oz / 120 g **13**

Cream cheese,
4 tsp **2**

Egg, 1 X large, poached,
boiled or fried, 2 oz / 60 g **7**

Butter / marg, 1½ tsp **0**
+ Peanut butter, 1½ tsp **2**

Banana, 1 med **3**

Baked Beans,
½ cup / 4.3 oz / 130 g **6**

Corn, kernels or creamed,
3.3 oz / 100 g **3**

Cheese, 1 slice,
0.6 oz / 20 g **5**

Avocado, ¹⁄₃, 2 oz / 60 g **1**

Yogurt, light or low fat plain,
6.7 oz / 200 g **15**

Yogurt, flavored, low fat,
4 oz / 120 g **4**

Ground beef,
2 oz / 55 g **11**

Hot fat free milk drink^,
6.7 fl oz / 200 ml **6**

Fat free milk^,
6.7 fl oz / 200 ml **7**

> **BAND TIP** Ensure drinks are taken a few minutes prior to solid food – the thicker the drink, the longer the delay.
> Please note that thin liquids are unlikely to be as satisfying as solid food.

Free foods (< 20 Cals / < 85 kJ)

* For more 'Free food' serves refer to Appendix 3

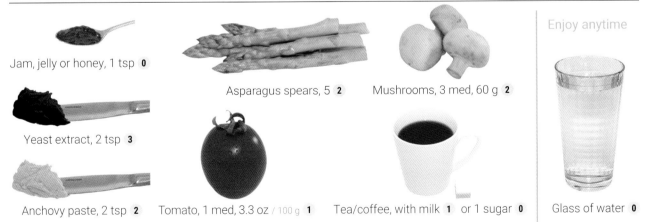

Jam, jelly or honey, 1 tsp **0**

Asparagus spears, 5 **2**

Mushrooms, 3 med, 60 g **2**

Enjoy anytime

Yeast extract, 2 tsp **3**

Anchovy paste, 2 tsp **2**

Tomato, 1 med, 3.3 oz / 100 g **1**

Tea/coffee, with milk **1** or 1 sugar **0**

Glass of water **0**

> **SLEEVE TIP** For sleeve owners, avoid drinking 45 minutes either side of a meal.

3 = Protein in grams. ⊜ = Contains probiotic bacteria. ^ = see p39 for equivalent plant milk.

Breakfast

Cereal, fruit and milk

The following cereal estimates contain 150 Calories / 630 kJ per serve. Compare your cereal to the nutritional criteria below and then identify the picture that most closely resembles your cereal to determine the recommended volume. Some volumes may be more suited to those who had their surgery some time ago, so choose a cereal with a volume you can consume or halve the volume using the ingredient combination listed below. If constipation is a problem, ensure you include the optional fibre component.

Meal components

Cals / kJ	Milk (50 Cals / 210 kJ)	Fruit (25 Cals / 105 kJ)	Cereal (150 Cals / 630 kJ)	Free (optional) (<20 Cals / 85kJ)
225 Cals / 945 kJ	1	1	1	1
Or 225 Cals / 945 kJ	2	2	½	1

Cereal Criteria

Because cereals have varying serving sizes listed on the pack, for the assessment of whether a cereal is healthy enough to consume everyday I recommend the CalorieKing app in the US and Australia or My Fitness Pal in the UK. Choose your cereal, enter a serve size of 100g and check the following criteria. Some countries may indicate the nutritional data for a 100g serve on the label.

1. Less than 14 g / 100 g sugar If no or very little fruit content **OR** Less than 28 g / 100 g of sugar if it contains significant fruit*
2. More than 8 g / 100 g fibre
3. Less than 4 g / 100 g saturated fat

* Considered to be 25% or more fruit content.

If you have diabetes, choose cereals that meet all 3 criteria, for general health ensure cereals meet at least 2 of the criteria listed.

Milk mini serves (50 Cals / 210 kJ)

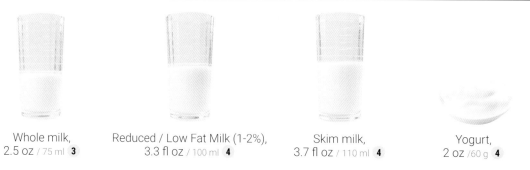

Whole milk, 2.5 oz / 75 ml **3**

Reduced / Low Fat Milk (1-2%), 3.3 fl oz / 100 ml **4**

Skim milk, 3.7 fl oz / 110 ml **4**

Yogurt, 2 oz /60 g **4**

Mini fruit serves (25 Cals / 105 kJ)

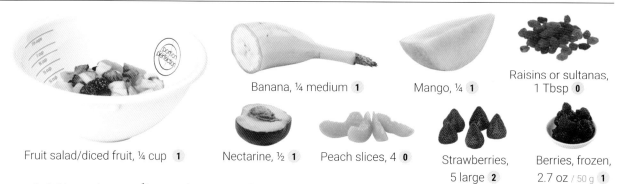

Banana, ¼ medium **1**

Mango, ¼ **1**

Raisins or sultanas, 1 Tbsp **0**

Fruit salad/diced fruit, ¼ cup **1**

Nectarine, ½ **1**

Peach slices, 4 **0**

Strawberries, 5 large **2**

Berries, frozen, 2.7 oz / 50 g **1**

For more fruit ideas, choose a ½ serve from Appendix 1 on page 112.

3 = Protein in grams.

Breakfast

Cereal, fruit and milk *continued*

After determining the suitability of your cereal choice, then use the guide below to recognise your cereal type.

1 serve = ¼ cup natural or toasted granola

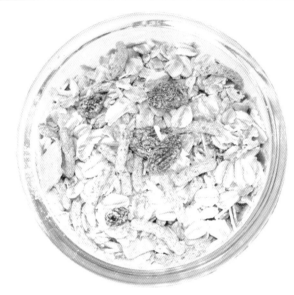

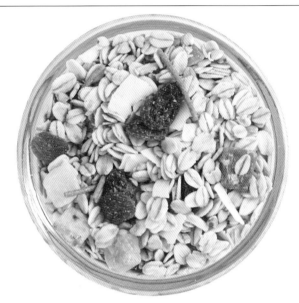

Natural Granola **4**

Toasted Granola **4**

1 serve = ½ cup (or 1.3 oz / 35 g packet) raw oats or clusters

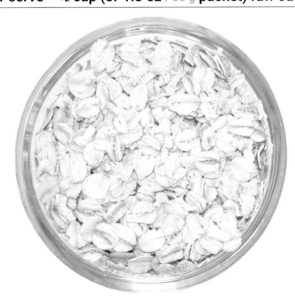

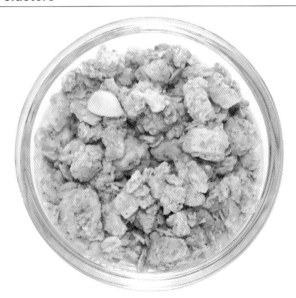

Raw Wholegrain or Steel Cut Oats **5**

Cluster Cereal **3**

Note: For oat pouches, look for 30-45g steel cut or wholegrain varieties.

3 = Protein in grams.

Continued over >

Breakfast

Cereal, fruit and milk *continued*

1 serve = ¾ cup mixed cereals or bran

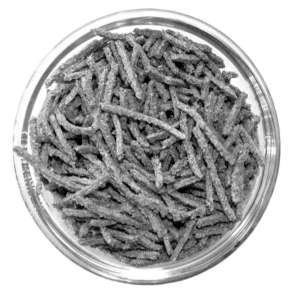

Processed Bran **7**

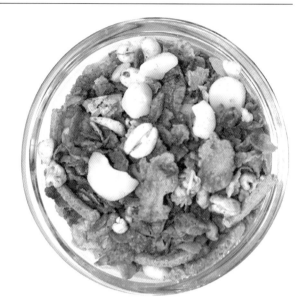

Fruit, Flakes and Nuts **4**

1 serve = 1 cup light or flaky cereals

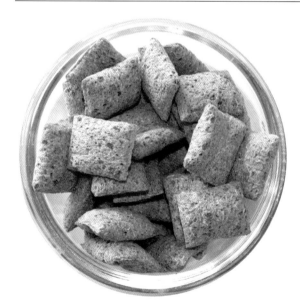

Light Cereals **4**

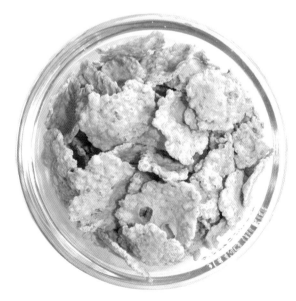

Flakes **5**

3 = Protein in grams.

Breakfast

Cereal, fruit and milk *continued*

1 serve = 1 cup *continued*

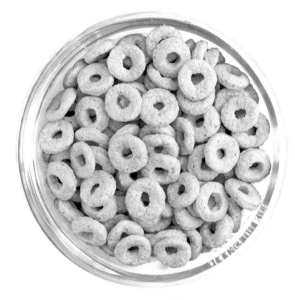

Loops **4**

2 large or 16 mini breakfast bix

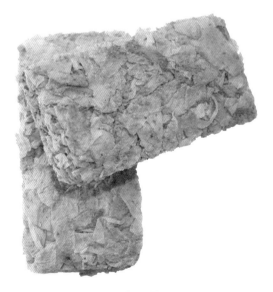

Weetabix **5**

Free Food – 1 Tbsp bran

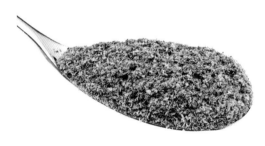

Bran – Oatbran, Psyllium, Wheatgerm, Unprocessed Bran **1**

3 = Protein in grams.

Breakfast
Yogurt and fruit

Meal components

Cals / kJ	Yogurt (200 Cals / 840 kJ)	Mini Fruit (25 Cals / 105 kJ)
225 Cals / 945 kJ	1	1
Or 225 Cals / 945 kJ	1/2	4

For example: 6.7 oz / 200 g tub of reduced fat flavored yogurt + ¼ cup fruit salad *Or* 3.3 oz / 100 g reduced fat flavored yogurt + a whole banana

Yogurt (200 Cals / 840 kJ)

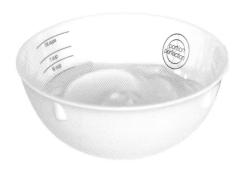

Greek style, ½ cup **8**

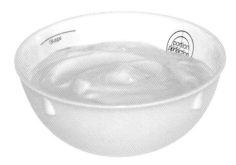

Greek style, no fat, 1 cup **17**

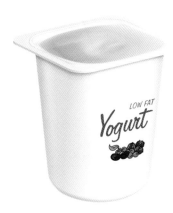

Low fat flavored yogurt, ⅔ cup, 6.7 oz / 200 g **10**

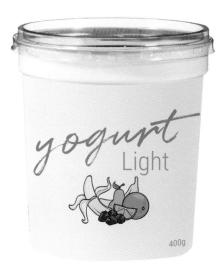

Low fat, art sw (light) yogurt, 1½ cups, 13.3 oz / 400 g **20**

Note: The 400g light yogurt is shown for reference and is likely to be too large a volume.

3 = Protein in grams.

Breakfast

Yogurt and fruit *continued*

Mini fruit serves (25 Cals / 105 kJ**)** More fruit serves appear in Appendix 1.

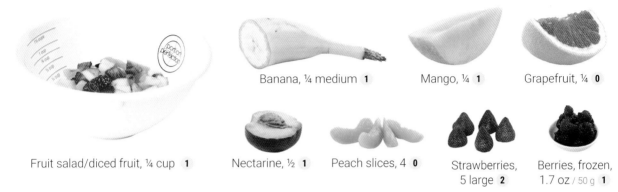

Banana, ¼ medium **1**   Mango, ¼ **1**   Grapefruit, ¼ **0**

Fruit salad/diced fruit, ¼ cup **1**   Nectarine, ½ **1**   Peach slices, 4 **0**   Strawberries, 5 large **2**   Berries, frozen, 1.7 oz / 50 g **1**

For more fruit ideas, choose a 1/2 serve from Appendix 1 on page 112.

"For those who have trouble eating solid food of a morning, choose pureed fruit and yogurt or a smoothie for the best start to the day."

3 = Protein in grams.

Breakfast

Smoothie

A smoothie can be constructed from fruit, milk or juice and either low fat ice cream or low fat yogurt and some fibre can be a great addition too. The thicker the better for sleeve and bypass owners and those with a loose band. Some band owners may need a thinner consistency. Another easy substitute is a packaged protein shake containing 20-30g protein and approx 200 Cals, eg., Premier Protein.

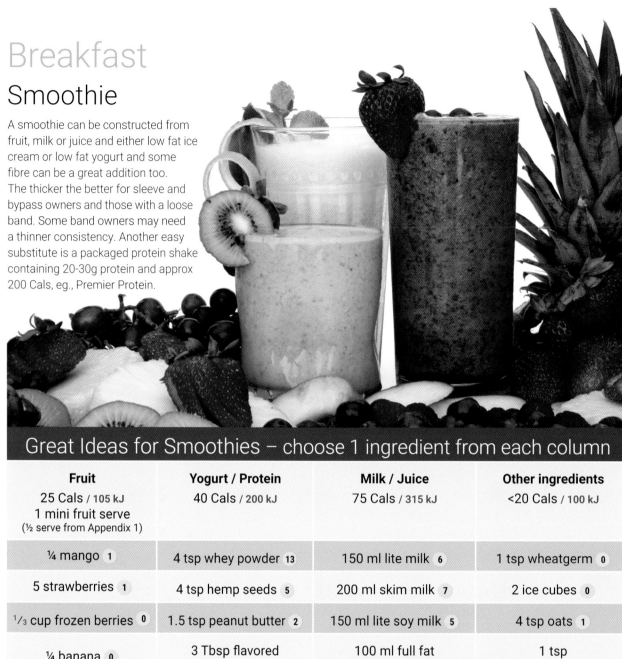

Great Ideas for Smoothies – choose 1 ingredient from each column

Fruit 25 Cals / 105 kJ 1 mini fruit serve (½ serve from Appendix 1)	Yogurt / Protein 40 Cals / 200 kJ	Milk / Juice 75 Cals / 315 kJ	Other ingredients <20 Cals / 100 kJ
¼ mango **1**	4 tsp whey powder **13**	150 ml lite milk **6**	1 tsp wheatgerm **0**
5 strawberries **1**	4 tsp hemp seeds **5**	200 ml skim milk **7**	2 ice cubes **0**
⅓ cup frozen berries **0**	1.5 tsp peanut butter **2**	150 ml lite soy milk **5**	4 tsp oats **1**
¼ banana **0**	3 Tbsp flavored yogurt **2**	100 ml full fat coffee flavored milk **3**	1 tsp psyllium husks **0**
1 pineapple slice **0**	4 tsp tasteless collagen powder **15**	150 ml reduced fat, low lactose milk **5**	1 tsp chia seeds **1**
½ cup kale or spinach **1**	4 tsp rice or soy protein powder* **9**	150 ml carrot and orange juice **0**	75 ml coconut water **0**
4 peach slices **0**	4 Tbsp Siggi's yogurt **5**	100 ml coconut milk **1**	1 tsp flaxseed meal **1**
½ kiwi fruit **0**	4 Tbsp natural yogurt **3**	200 ml almond milk **1**	Water **0**

TIP Choose a local milk fortified with additional Vitamin D. 1 mini fruit serve, 3 Tbsp yogurt or ice cream + 5 fl oz / 150 ml milk.

3 = Protein in grams.

Breakfast

Omelette

An omelette is a great way to get some protein into your diet. There's endless combinations of flavors you can create.

Start with **+** 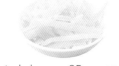 Then add a selection of 3 serves from the following 'free' foods.

1 X large egg, 2 oz / 60 g **7**   Grated cheese, .85 oz / 25 g **7**

Free foods (< 20 Cals / < 85 kJ)

* For more 'free food' serves refer to Appendix 3

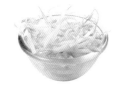

Bean sprouts, 1 oz / 35 g **1**

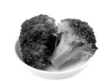

Broccoli, 1 oz / 30 g **1**

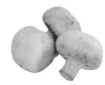

Mushrooms, 2 oz / 60 g **2**

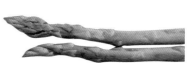

Asparagus spears, 2 **1**

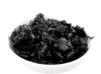

Spinach, chopped finely, 1 oz / 30 g **1**

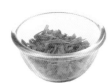

Grated carrot, ¼ cup, 1 oz / 30 g **0**

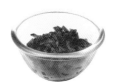

Capsicum/bell pepper, ¼ cup, 0.2 oz / 5 g **0**

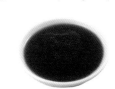

Soya, Worcestershire, BBQ or tomato sauce, 1 Tbsp **0**

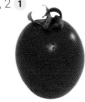

Tomato, 3.3 oz / 100 g **1**

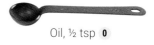

Oil, ½ tsp **0**

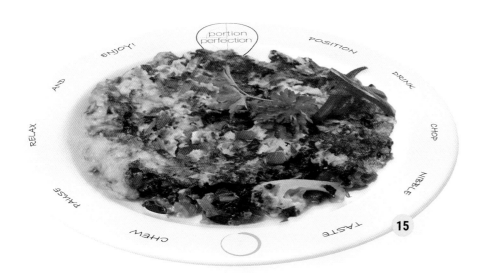

Actual size of circle on plate

 TIP Chop all ingredients small enough to fit through the small circle on the rim of the plate above.

3 = Protein in grams.

Breakfast

Legumes

These are true super foods and well tolerated by band and sleeve owners alike. Beans and lentils contain the protein of meat, the starch of grains and the nutrients of vegetables. They don't have a strong flavor, but absorb the flavors of ingredients surrounding them. Take the time to experiment with new recipes.

Meal components

Cals / kJ	Beans (100 Cals / 420 kJ)	Bread/Toast (100 Cals / 420 kJ)
200 Cals / 840 kJ	1	1
200 Cals / 840 kJ	2	0

1 bean serve (100 Cals / 420 kJ)

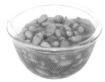

TIP There's some great legume recipes in the 4 Week Weight Loss Menu Plan.

½ cup baked beans, chickpeas, kidney beans or bean salad **6**

1 bread serve (100 Cals / 420 kJ)

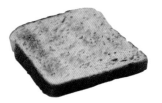 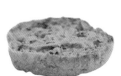 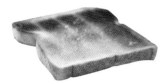 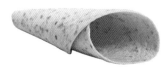

Wholegrain bread, 1 slice, 1 oz / 30 g **3**

English muffin, ½ wholegrain **4**

Low GI white bread, 1 slice, 1 oz / 30 g **3**

Tortilla, whole wheat or grain, 1 small, 1 oz / 30g **3**

TIP Canned beans are just as nutritious and more convenient than soaking your own.

TIP Dried lentils don't need soaking. Just boil in stock.

TIP Red lentils take about the same amount of time as rice to cook and almost disintegrate into wet dishes adding valuable texture and protein.

3 = Protein in grams.

"Become familiar with Beans, Peas and Lentils."

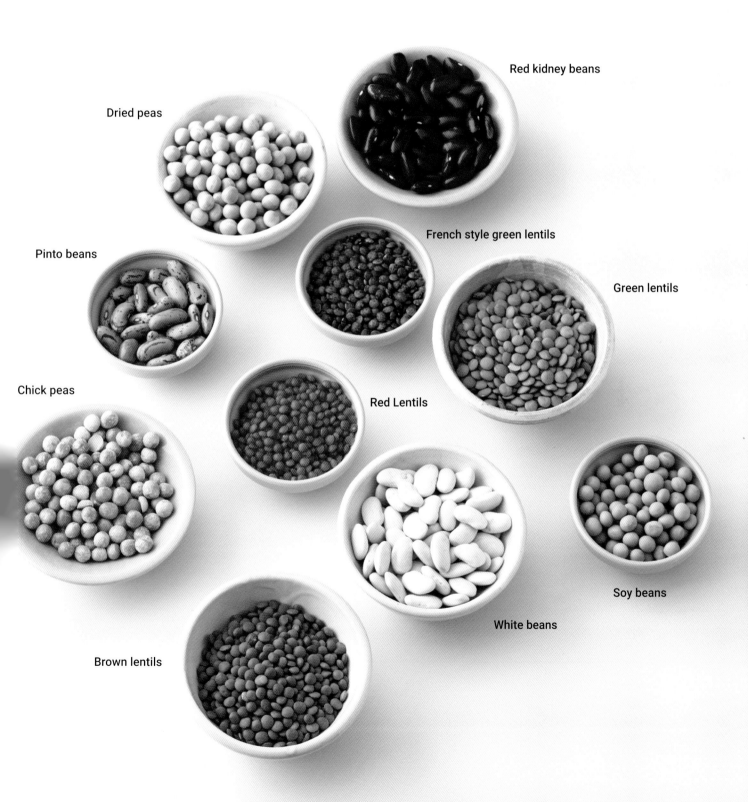

Dried peas

Red kidney beans

Pinto beans

French style green lentils

Green lentils

Chick peas

Red Lentils

White beans

Soy beans

Brown lentils

"What you choose for lunch
can influence those
mid-afternoon munchies."

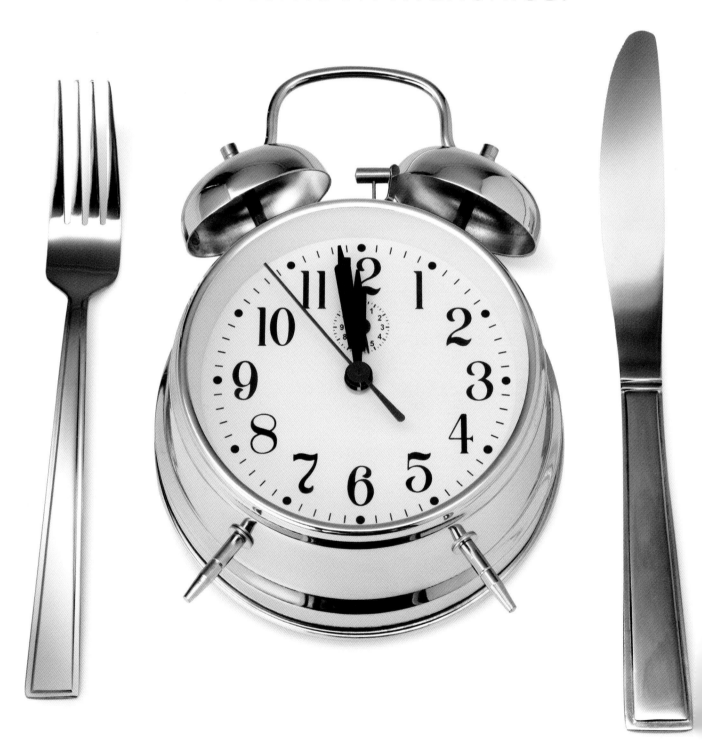

lunch

Lunch is often taken on the run or skipped altogether. What you choose for lunch can influence those mid-afternoon munchies. So you want to get it right most of the time. Lack of food earlier in the day may contribute to excessive intake in the evening and inadvertently stretching and increasing the capacity of the smaller stomach pouch.

Whether you're preparing food at home or dining out, the marker of a good choice is the vegetable content. If your usual choice consists only of bread or potato and meat it'll weigh you down for the afternoon. Choose combinations of wholegrains, protein foods and salad or vegetables.

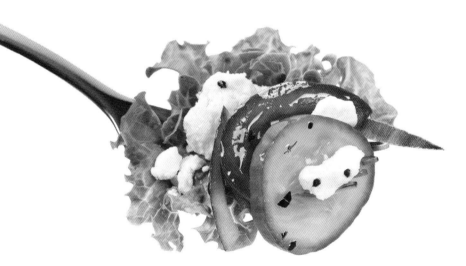

everyday menu   page
Sandwiches 72
Soup 74
Salads 75
Snack Style or Bento Box Lunch 76
Sashimi and Sushi 80
Kebabs/Gyros 81
Burgers 82

occasional menu   page
Chicken Nuggets and Fries 83
Fish & Chips 83

Add your own favourites by calculating a 200-250 Cal / 840 kJ-950 kJ serve from *Calorieking* or *My Fitness Pal*.

Everyday Lunch
Sandwiches

Many people find that bread causes problems due to its doughy texture after bariatric surgery. If this is a problem for you, toast the bread, or choose grainy crispbreads. Follow the guide to construct an open sandwich or ½ of a traditional sandwich. When eating out in the US make sure you request NO CRISPS to avoid sabotaging your healthy choice.

Meal components

Cals / kJ	Bread (100 Cals / 420 kJ)	Protein (50 Cals / 210 kJ)	Mini Add Ons (50 Cals / 210 kJ)	Salad and free foods (< 20 Cals / 84 kJ)
220 Cals / 924 kJ	1	1	1	1

Breads (100 Cals / 420 kJ)

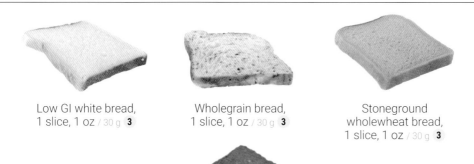

Low GI white bread, 1 slice, 1 oz / 30 g **3**

Wholegrain bread, 1 slice, 1 oz / 30 g **3**

Stoneground wholewheat bread, 1 slice, 1 oz / 30 g **3**

Wholegrain crackers, 0.8 oz / 25g **3**

Rye crispbread, 0.8 oz / 25 g **2**

Pumpernickel bread, 1 slice, 1.7 oz / 50 g **3**

Grainy corn/rice cakes, 4 **3**

Tortilla, whole wheat or grain, 1 small, 1 oz / 30g **3**

 TIP Higher fibre breads and cereals are also higher in other nutrients such as folate, thiamine and riboflavin.

Protein (50 Cals / 210 kJ)

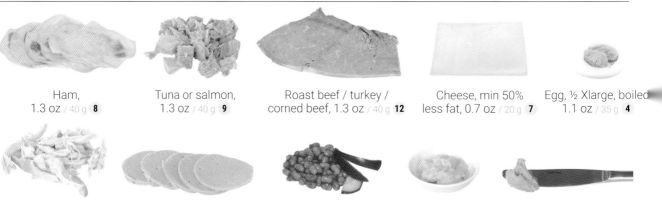

Ham, 1.3 oz / 40 g **8**

Tuna or salmon, 1.3 oz / 40 g **9**

Roast beef / turkey / corned beef, 1.3 oz / 40 g **12**

Cheese, min 50% less fat, 0.7 oz / 20 g **7**

Egg, ½ Xlarge, boiled 1.1 oz / 35 g **4**

Chicken, 1 oz / 30 g **7**

Vegetarian sausage, 1 oz / 30 g **4**

Baked beans, ½ can, 2 oz / 65 g **3**

Hummus, 1.3 oz / 16 g **1**

Peanut butter, 1.5 tsp **2**

3 = Protein in grams.

Everyday Lunch

Sandwiches *continued*

Mini Add Ons (50 Cals / 210 kJ**)** – see Appendix 2 for full list

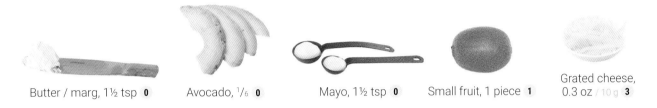

Butter / marg, 1½ tsp **0**   Avocado, ¹/₆ **0**   Mayo, 1½ tsp **0**   Small fruit, 1 piece **1**   Grated cheese, 0.3 oz / 10 g **3**

Salad (< 20 Cals / 84 kJ**)**

Any combination of the following:

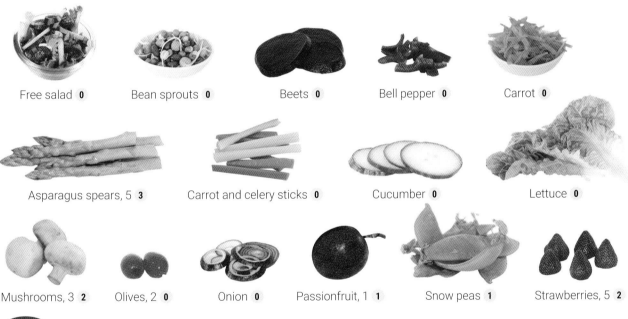

Free salad **0**   Bean sprouts **0**   Beets **0**   Bell pepper **0**   Carrot **0**

Asparagus spears, 5 **3**   Carrot and celery sticks **0**   Cucumber **0**   Lettuce **0**

Mushrooms, 3 **2**   Olives, 2 **0**   Onion **0**   Passionfruit, 1 **1**   Snow peas **1**   Strawberries, 5 **2**

 Ensure 'fibrous' or 'stringy' vegetables such as celery are chopped small enough.

"The value of bariatric surgery is that you effectively have a whole new stomach and an opportunity to maintain a tiny appetite."

3 = Protein in grams.

Everyday Lunch

Soups

Choose thick soups, with added protein in the form of meat, chicken, fish or legumes, such as a minestrone soup (see below).

1.5 cups soup = 200 Cals / 840 kJ

7

Minestrone Soup Recipe

Ingredients

400g canned diced peeled tomatoes

2 carrots, diced

2 celery sticks with leaves, chopped

3 pontiac potatoes, peeled, chopped

200g piece jap or butternut pumpkin, deseeded, peeled, chopped

1 onion, chopped

1 large garlic clove, crushed

1 tsp dried or 1 Tbsp fresh chopped oregano leaves

7 cups water

2 large zucchini/courgette, chopped

40g (1/4 cup) small macaroni

400g canned red kidney beans, rinsed, drained

1/2 cup firmly packed roughly chopped fresh continental parsley

freshly ground black pepper

Extra 1 tsp extra virgin olive oil and 2 tsp of parmesan per serve.

Method

1. Place the tomatoes, carrots, celery, potatoes, pumpkin, onion, garlic and oregano in a large saucepan.

2. Add the water, stir and bring to the boil over medium-high heat. Reduce heat and simmer, almost covered, for 45 minutes.

3. Add the zucchini/courgette and macaroni, and cook, stirring occasionally, for 10 minutes. Stir in the beans and cook for a further 5 minutes or until the zucchini/courgette and pasta are tender.

4. Stir in the parsley and pepper. Ladle into serving bowls.

5. Drizzle 1 tsp of the olive oil and 2 tsp of parmesan over each serve and enjoy!

6. Freeze additional 1.5 cup serves in snap lock bags.

Makes 10 x 1.5 Cup serves – freeze additional serves

"Canned soups can be a great option. Look for a chunky meat and vegetable soup."

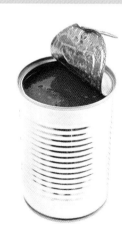

3 = Protein in grams.

Everyday Lunch
Salads

Meal components

Cals / kJ	Protein 50 Cals / 210 kJ	Salad < 20 Cals / 84 kJ	Mini Add Ons 50 Cals / 210 kJ
220 Cals / 924 kJ	3	½ Cup	1

Protein (50 Cals / 210 kJ)

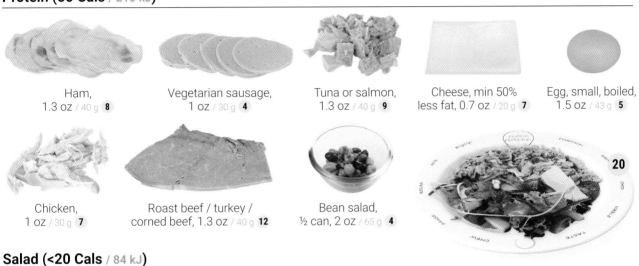

Ham,
1.3 oz / 40 g **8**

Vegetarian sausage,
1 oz / 30 g **4**

Tuna or salmon,
1.3 oz / 40 g **9**

Cheese, min 50%
less fat, 0.7 oz / 20 g **7**

Egg, small, boiled,
1.5 oz / 43 g **5**

Chicken,
1 oz / 30 g **7**

Roast beef / turkey /
corned beef, 1.3 oz / 40 g **12**

Bean salad,
½ can, 2 oz / 65 g **4**

20

Salad (<20 Cals / 84 kJ)

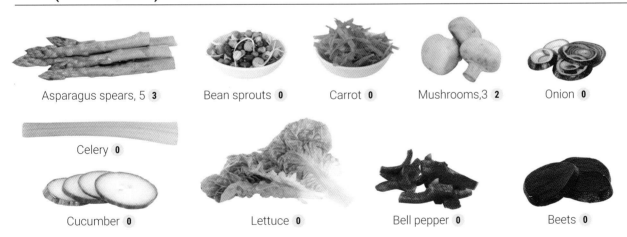

Asparagus spears, 5 **3**

Bean sprouts **0**

Carrot **0**

Mushrooms,3 **2**

Onion **0**

Celery **0**

Cucumber **0**

Lettuce **0**

Bell pepper **0**

Beets **0**

1 Mini Add On (50 Cals / 210 kJ)

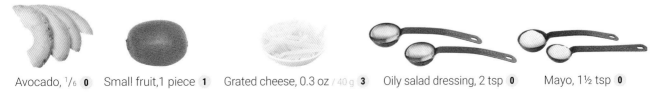

Avocado, ¹/₆ **0**   Small fruit,1 piece **1**   Grated cheese, 0.3 oz / 40 g **3**   Oily salad dressing, 2 tsp **0**   Mayo, 1½ tsp **0**

3 = Protein in grams.

Everyday Lunch

Snack Style or Bento Box Lunch

Bento boxes are a meal for one with separate spaces for each meal component. They make for a fun, snack style lunch with great opportunity for variety in flavours and textures.

Meal components

Cals / kJ	Protein – Meat / Dairy / Alternatives (50 Cals / 210 kJ)	Carbohydrate – Bread / Fruit (50 Cals / 210 kJ)	Fat – Oils (50 Cals / 210 kJ)	Free Foods – Veg / Salad (20 Cals / 84kJ)
220 Cals / 924 kJ	2	1	1	1

Protein (50 Cals / 210 kJ) *2 serves*

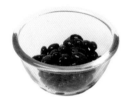
Baked, black or kidney beans or chickpeas, ¼ cup **3**

Cheese, 50% less fat, 20 g **7**

Cheese, full fat, ½ slice or grated, 10 g **3**

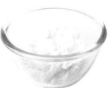
Cottage cheese, ¼ cup **8**

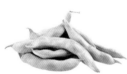
Edamame beans, shelled, 30 g **4**

Egg, 1 small or ½ extra large **4**

Falafel ball, 1 x 25 g **1**

Feta or Camembert cheese, 10 g **2**

Fish cake, 1 small, 40 g **5**

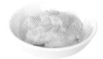
Hummus, 1 Tbsp **1**

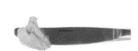
Peanut butter, 1.5 tsp **2**

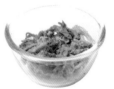
Pulled / shredded meat, e.g., chicken, pork, beef, 40 g **9** to **12**

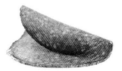
Salami, thin slice, 15 g **3**

Seeds, Hemp, 1 Tbsp **5**

Seeds, sunflower or pepita, 1 Tbsp **3**

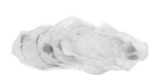
Shaved meat, e.g., ham **8**, pastrami **9**, turkey **12**, 40 g

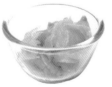
Salmon, smoked, 50 g **11**

Tofu or tempeh, 35 g **4**

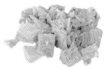
Tuna or salmon, ½ can, 40 g **9**

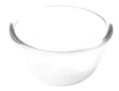
Yogurt, ¼ cup **3**

3 = Protein in grams.

Everyday Lunch

Snack Style or Bento Box Lunch *continued*

Carbohydrate (50 Cals / 210 kJ) *1 serve*

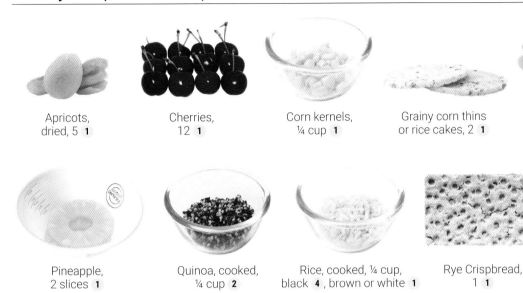

Apricots, dried, 5 **1**

Cherries, 12 **1**

Corn kernels, ¼ cup **1**

Grainy corn thins or rice cakes, 2 **1**

Grapes, small bunch, 100 g **1**

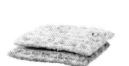

Pineapple, 2 slices **1**

Quinoa, cooked, ¼ cup **2**

Rice, cooked, ¼ cup, black **4**, brown or white **1**

Rye Crispbread, 1 **1**

Raisins, 15 g **0**

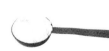
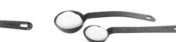
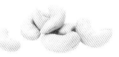

Sushi, 1 piece, 30 g **2**

Tortilla, ½ small, toasted, 15 g **1**

Triscuits, 2 **1**

Wholegrain bread, ½ slice, 15 g **2**

Wholegrain rice snacks, 6 **1**

Fats (50 Cals / 210 kJ) *1 serve*

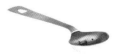
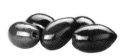

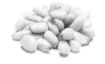
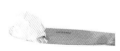

Avocado, ¹⁄₆, 30 g **0**

Coconut, 1 Tbsp, 8 g **0**

Cream cheese, 2 tsp **1** or 1 Tbsp light **2**

Mayo, 1½ tsp **0**

Nuts, e.g., almonds or cashews, 7, 10 g **2**

Oil, e.g., olive, argan, flax 1 tsp **0**

Olives, 5 **0**

Pesto **1** or tahini **2** 2 tsp

Seeds, e.g., pinenuts, 1 Tbsp, 10 g **2**

Spread, 1½ tsp **0**

3 = Protein in grams.

Everyday Lunch

Snack Style or Bento Box Lunch *continued*

Free Foods (< 20 Cals / 84 kJ**)** *1 serve*

Bean sprouts **0**

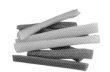

Carrot and celery sticks **0**

Cherry tomatoes, 5 **0**

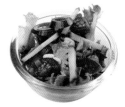

Free salad **0**

Mushrooms **1**

Passionfruit, 1 **1**

Pickled ginger **0**

Sauce – vinegar, soy,
teriyaki, tomato, 1 Tbsp **0**

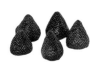

Strawberries, 5 **1**

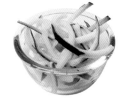

Zucchini/Courgette
or carrot spirals, **0**

"Consuming oil with vegetables increases the absorption of a range of nutrients – plan for a dressing of our culinary argan oil with balsamic vinegar for the added benefit of improved skin elasticity."

3 = Protein in grams.

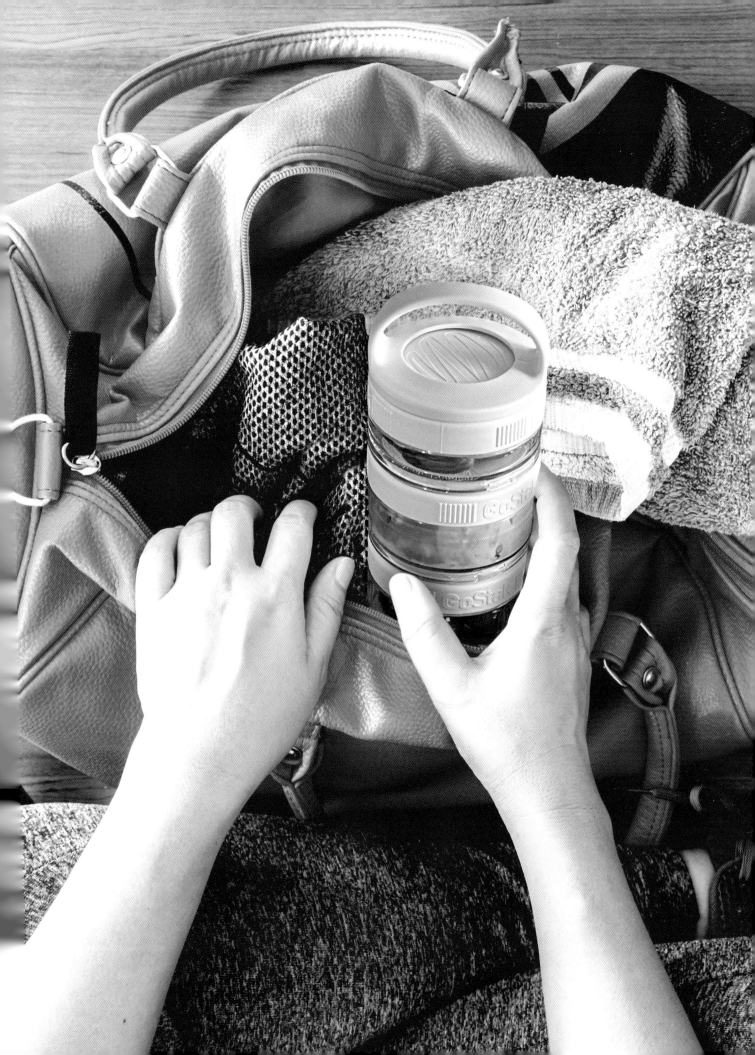

Everyday Lunch

Sashimi and Sushi

Sashimi and sushi are becoming very convenient lunch choices. They're nice and petite, so you only expect to eat a small volume. Most sushi is relatively low GI.

200 Cals / 840 kJ

Sashimi, 4 oz / 120 g

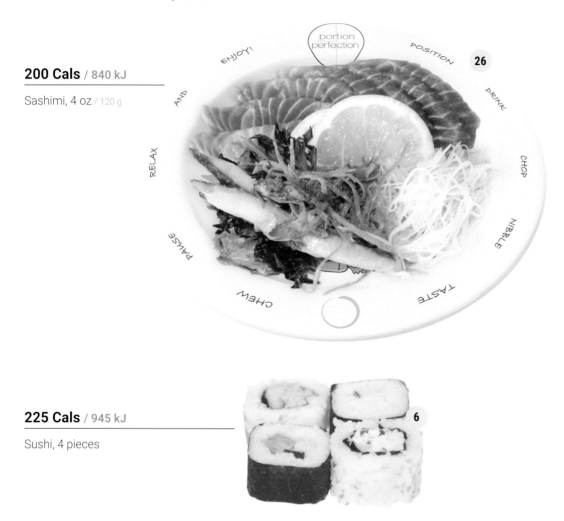

225 Cals / 945 kJ

Sushi, 4 pieces

"Bariatric surgeries work because they result in satisfaction from smaller portions of food."

3 = Protein in grams.

Everyday Lunch

Doner Kebab/Gyros

A kebab is a convenient option when out and about. Ask for it to be cut in half so you can share or clearly see your stopping point.

225 Cals / 945 kJ

½ a standard sized meat kebab (no cheese), with low fat sauce eg. Barbecue or tomato

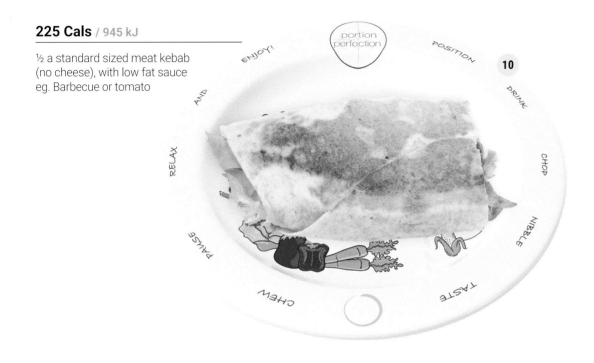

Partner perspective

"I used to find myself eating my own meal and then my partners leftovers. Now, if for example, we wanted kebabs we'd each eat half and I'd add a fruit salad or a cappucino to make the calorie intake right for me."

Sue

3 = Protein in grams.

Everyday Lunch

Burger

With a bit of planning a burger or a toasted turkish or foccacia can be a good choice. Either choose to eat half the burger or just the insides. Choose options with lots of salad and ask them to hold the fries. Choose burgers without the extras such as bacon, cheese or egg and don't forget to have a drink of water beforehand.

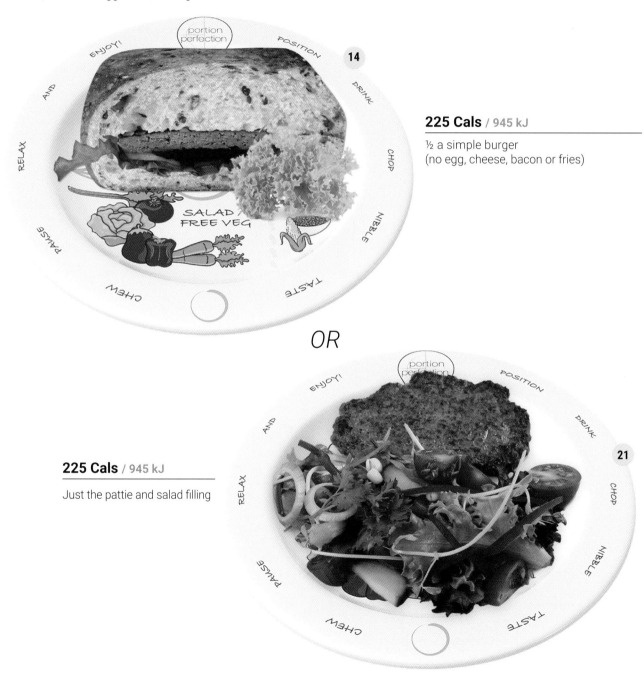

225 Cals / 945 kJ

½ a simple burger
(no egg, cheese, bacon or fries)

OR

225 Cals / 945 kJ

Just the pattie and salad filling

3 = Protein in grams.

Occasional Lunch

If you should find yourself faced with fried foods, focus your attention on the protein. Let the fries go cold so they're not so appealing and portion off the amount you see below to enjoy. Look for opportunities to add some salad.

Nuggets and fries **200 Cals** / 840 kJ

3 nuggets + 3 large or 7 small fries

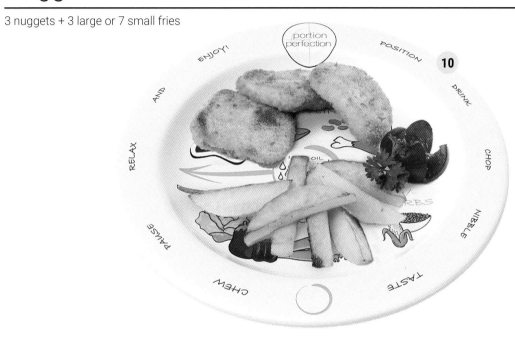

Fish and fries **200 Cals** / 840 kJ

½ piece of battered fish + 3 large or 7 small fries

3 = Protein in grams.

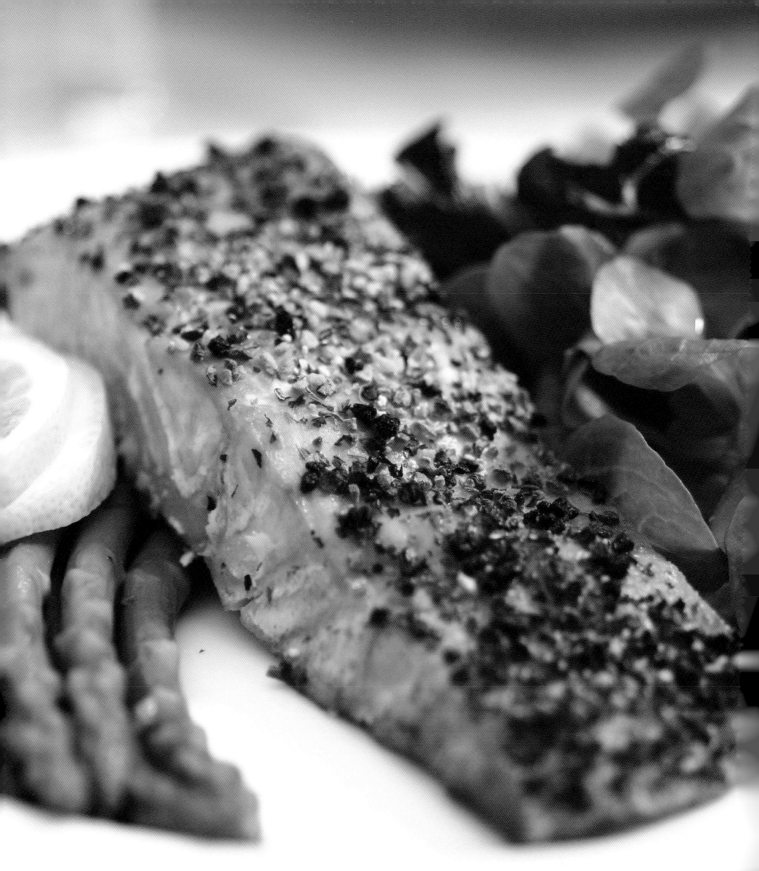

"Listen for that moment of satisfaction."

dinner

Dinners each contain 200 – 250 Cals when served appropriately on the plate. The protein and oil components of the plate contain around 180 Cals / 750 kJ. The free vegetable or salad component contains around 20 Cals / 84 kJ, so just choosing protein and free vegetables will supply approx 200 Cals / 840 kJ. (see diagram below).

By including carbohydrate in the small area delineated, the meal will total approximately 250 Cals / 1050 kJ.

The value of avoiding the carbohydrate at dinner and just choosing protein and a larger serve of green and low starch vegetables is a larger dose of nutrients, specifically folate and the protective factors found in vegetables.

Skipping the carbohydrate does also mean dropping your daily calorie intake by a further 50 Calories / 220 kJ which may provide a small added benefit to weekly weight loss.

If you take medication for diabetes then including the carbohydrate section is a must. For others it is optional, so seek the guidance of your dietitian if needed.

Remember to follow the wording around the outside of the plate to get the eating behaviours right. See page 32 for a full explanation of the terms.

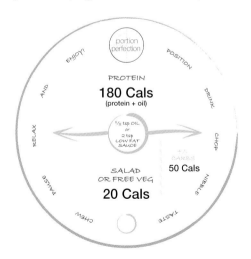

200 – 250 Cals / 840 – 1050 kJ

While it may look as though there are only 5 evening meal options represented here, the reality is that the options are endless. By varying the protein, vegetable, sauce and carbohydrate components, you create an endless array of meals that fit the ideal formula.

Look for meal ideas from your favourite recipe books. Choose recipes that use 1 fl oz / 30 ml or less of added fat for a recipe designed for 4 full sized serves.

Be prepared for leftovers. Cover and refrigerate leftovers straight away to avoid the temptation of eating more before "satisfaction" has set in.

Choose cookbooks loaded with illustrated, basic tasty recipes made from everyday ingredients. The best ones also have the nutritional breakdown of each recipe.

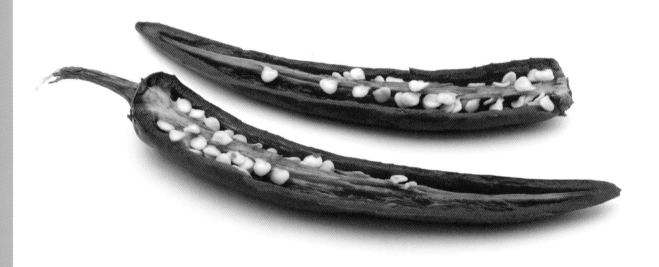

everyday menu   page
Bolognaise and salad 87
Roast meat and vegetables......................88
Fish, meat, chicken and salad...................89
Vegetarian...90
Beef and vegetable stir fry 91

occasional menu   page
Takeaway foods......................................92

Add your own favourites by calculating the appropriate serve from *Calorieking* or *My Fitness Pal.*

3 = Protein in grams.

Everyday Dinner
Bolognaise and salad

Ground meats are well tolerated by most. Choose the best quality ground meats or poultry possible and prepare according to your Mum's favourite recipe or consult a healthy cookbook for new ideas. Always serve with a green salad for the perfect meal.

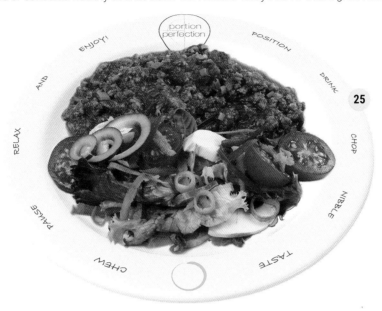

200 Cals / 840 kJ

Bolognaise and salad
(4 oz / 120 g raw weight ground meat)

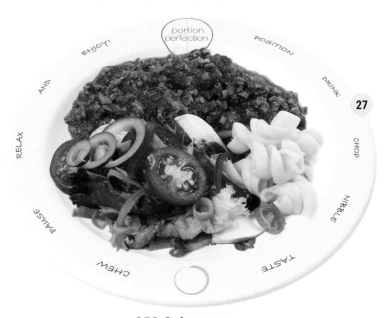

250 Cals / 1050 kJ

Bolognaise and salad with pasta
(4 oz / 120 g raw weight ground meat)

3 = Protein in grams.

Everyday Dinner
Roast meat and vegetables

Choose from chicken, turkey, beef, pork, lamb or fish. Meats can be marinated, grilled, barbecued or baked. Moist cooking methods are the best. Choose whether to include the carbohydrate (bread and potatoes) or add extra green vegetables to the steamer.

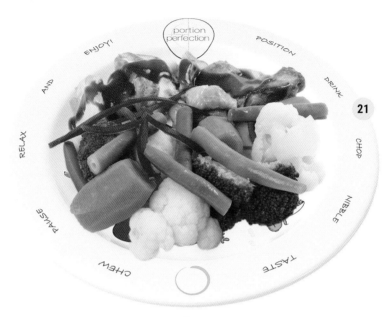

200 Cals / 840 kJ

Roast Chicken and vegetables

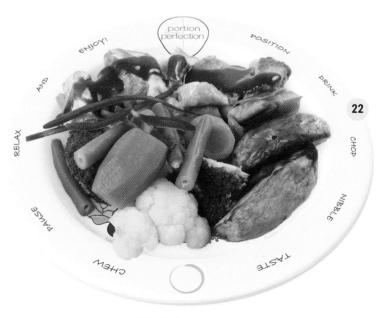

250 Cals / 1050 kJ

Roast Chicken and vegetables with yam and potato

3 = Protein in grams.

Everyday Dinner
Fish / meat / chicken and salad

Fish is very well tolerated after all bariatric surgeries. It is moist, tender, low in bad fats and can be cooked in a variety of ways. Choose cooking methods with small amounts of added fat and choose low fat sauces if desired. Fish is the perfect accompaniment to a green salad. Add Basmati rice, pasta, yam or corn for low GI carbohydrate.

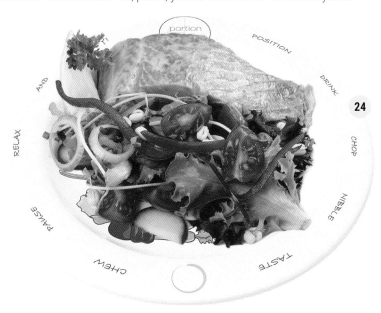

200 Cals / 840 kJ

Salmon steak and salad

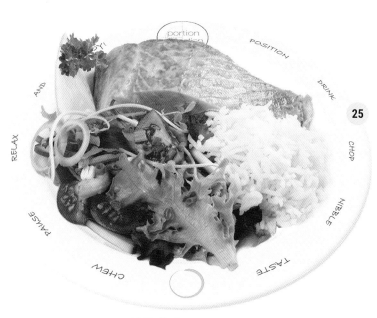

250 Cals / 1050 kJ

Salmon steak and salad with rice

3 = Protein in grams.

Everyday Dinner

Vegetarian

Legumes are one of the most versatile, cheap, nutritious and well tolerated foods after bariatric surgery. If you're unfamiliar with them, get hold of a good vegetarian cookbook to learn the ropes. The recipe for this chickpea casserole comes from the kitchen of my colleague Anna Rose and appears in Appendix 4. Chickpeas and all other legumes contain carbohydrate as well as protein, so even with diabetes there is no necessity to add extra, but cous cous goes nicely if you choose to add more.

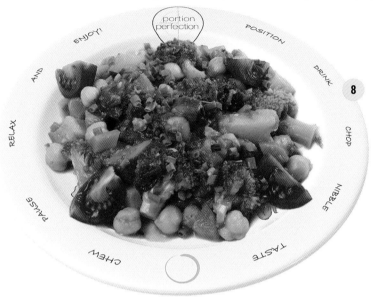

200 Cals / 840 kJ

Chickpea casserole

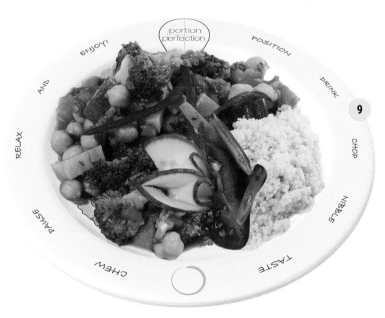

250 Cals / 1050 kJ

Chickpea casserole with cous cous

3 = Protein in grams.

Everyday Dinner
Beef and vegetable stir fry

RECIPE IDEA

A stir fry can be a great quick and easy meal. The colour, flavour and texture can be easily changed by varying the vegetables, the meat or the sauce. Cut meat across the grain and mix with oil instead of adding oil to the wok or pan. Ensure the pan is hot enough to evaporate a bead of water before adding meat. Cook in small batches and set aside while cooking the vegetables.

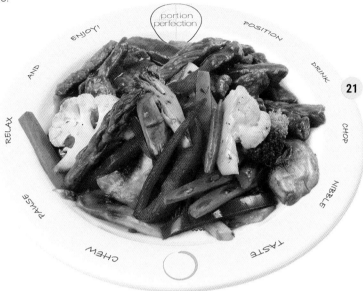

200 Cals / 840 kJ

Beef and vegetable stir fry

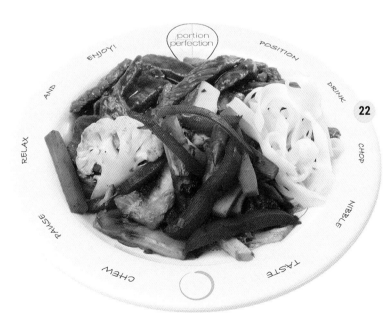

250 Cals / 1050 kJ

Beef and vegetable stir fry with noodles

3 = Protein in grams.

Occasional Dinner
Takeaway foods

Chinese

Chinese food is often fried before being stir fried. Choose meat and vegetable based meals rather than meat only dishes. Avoid choices with deep fried items as the appropriate portion size becomes smaller and less fulfilling. Jasmine rice is high GI, however even choosing steamed rice, rather than fried, would allow a slightly larger portion size for the Calories.

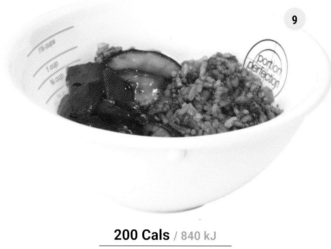

200 Cals / 840 kJ

2/3 Cup Chinese

Pizza

Choose 1 slice of thin and crispy style pizza with some vegetable toppings. Avoid stuffed crusts and extra meat or cheese.

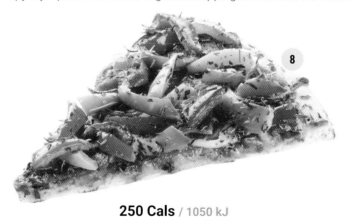

250 Cals / 1050 kJ

1 slice pizza

3 = Protein in grams.

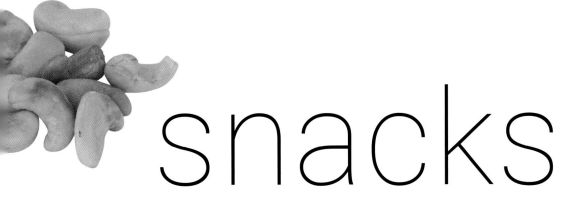

snacks

To snack or not to snack – ask your dietitian the question

My position is that snacks are best planned for – this way you can make them healthy most of the time. They help control appetite at meal times, keep metabolism ticking over and are a vital source of additional nutrients after bariatric surgery.

I recommend choosing a snack for mid morning, mid afternoon and supper from the vital snack list. The vital snack list includes fruit, nuts, vegetables and dairy as these contain critical nutrients for those on a very low Calorie intake. If you are in the weight loss phase, stick with these choices as they will provide optimum nutrition when intake is tightly limited.

Muesli bars, biscuits and other snacks containing lower levels of critical nutrients can be enjoyed twice per week as part of the occasional category. When you reach weight maintenance, if your weight doesn't naturally stabilise, you will be able to increase your Calorie intake and include more of these snacks.

Vital 100 Calorie snack menu*

Fruit 94
Nuts... 96
Vegetables and dip......................... 98
Dairy 100
Higher protein choices 103

Occasional 100 Calorie snack menu

Bars 105
Frozen desserts 106
Biscuits, cookies and crackers...107
Miscellaneous 108

* **All snacks selected for the 100 Cal** / 420 kJ **section contain 60 – 130 Cals** / 252 – 546 kJ.

Add your own favourites by calculating the appropriate serve from *Calorieking* or *My Fitness Pal*.

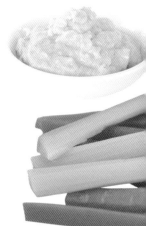

Vital Snacks
Fruit

Fruit is a perfect portion controlled snack. A 100 Cal / 420 kJ fruit snack generally consists of two small fruit serves or one large fruit serve. Fresh fruit may be more satisfying than dried fruit as one cup fresh fruit = approx ⅓ cup dried fruit.

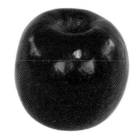

Apple, 1 large, 7 oz / 216 g **1**

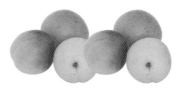

Apricots, 6 medium, total 6.7 oz / 200 g **2**

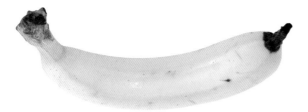

Banana, 1 medium, 6 oz / 170 g **3**

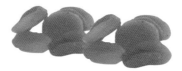

Dried apricots, 10, total 1 oz / 35 g **2**

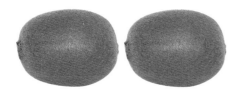

Kiwi fruit, 2 large, total 6.7 oz / 200 g **3**

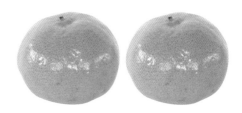

Mandarins, 2 large, total 6.7 oz / 200 g **2**

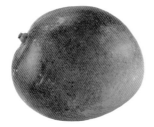

Mango, 1 small, total 6.7 oz / 200 g **2**

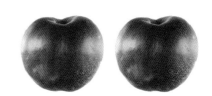

Nectarines, 2 medium, total 6.7 oz / 200 g **2**

3 = Protein in grams.

Vital Snacks

Fruit *continued*

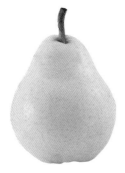

Pear, 1 large, 6.7 oz / 200 g **1**

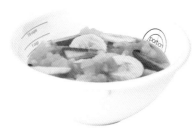

Fruit salad, 1 cup **2**

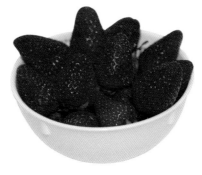

Strawberries, total 1 lb / 500 g **8**

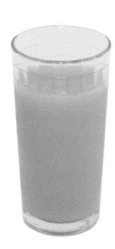

Various brands, Fruit juice,
6.7 fl oz / 200 ml **1**

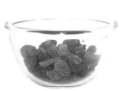

Dried fruit, 2 Tbsp,
1.3 oz / 40 g **1**

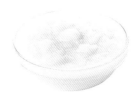

Applesauce,
½ cup, 4.7 oz / 140g **1**

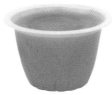

Fruit puree ½ cup, 4.3 oz / 130 g **0**

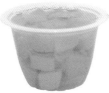

Canned fruit, ½ cup, 4.7 oz / 140 g **1**

 TIP Refer to Appendix 1 for more ideas.

3 = Protein in grams.

Vital Snacks
Nuts and seeds

Nuts are fairly concentrated in Calories due to their healthy oil content, but be aware that this means the portion size needs to be small compared to other foods. Nuts may be a perfect, quick and simple solution to the snack times when you are not looking for bulk.

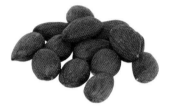

Almonds, 14,
0.7 oz / 20 g **4**

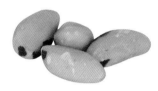

Brazil Nuts, 4,
0.7 oz / 20 g **3**

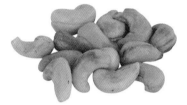

Cashews, 14,
0.7 oz / 20 g **4**

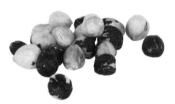

Hazelnuts, 20,
0.5 oz / 15 g **3**

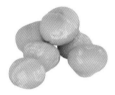

Macadamias, 6,
0.7 oz / 20 g **2**

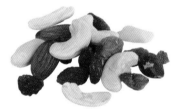

Mixed Fruit & Nuts,
0.7 oz / 20 g **2**

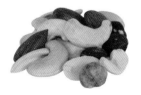

Mixed nuts,
0.7 oz / 18 g **3**

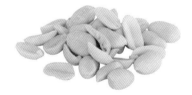

Peanuts, 36 halves,
0.7 oz / 18 g **5**

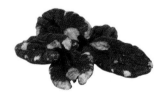

Pecans, 5,
0.7 oz / 20 g **2**

3 = Protein in grams.

Vital Snacks

Nuts and seeds *continued*

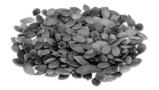

Pepitas, 2 Tbsp,
0.7 oz / 20 g **6**

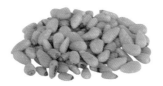

Pinenuts, 2 Tbsp,
0.7 oz / 18 g **3**

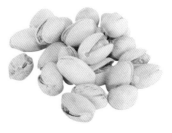

Pistachios, 25,
0.7 oz / 20 g shelled **4**

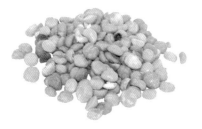

Roasted chickpeas, ¼ cup,
0.8 oz / 25 g **5**

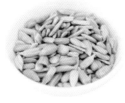

Sunflower seeds, 1.5 Tbsp,
0.7 oz / 18 g **4**

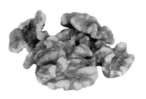

Walnuts, 6,
0.7 oz / 20 g **3**

TIP

You'll note that most serves here are around 20 g which is roughly the amount that fits into a cupped palm.

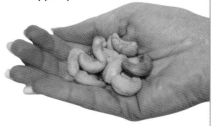

3 = Protein in grams.

Vital Snacks
Vegetables and dip

Choose one vegetable serve and 1 dip portion.

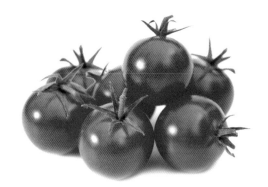

Cherry tomatoes, 7 **2**

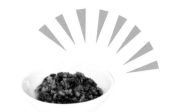

1 Tbsp oily dip **2**

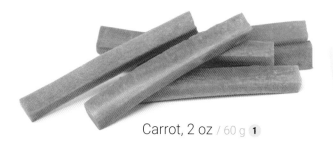

Carrot, 2 oz / 60 g **1**

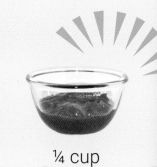

¼ cup
salsa **1** or tzatziki **1**

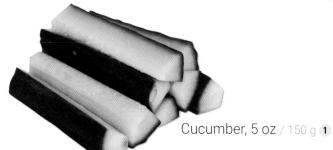

Cucumber, 5 oz / 150 g **1**

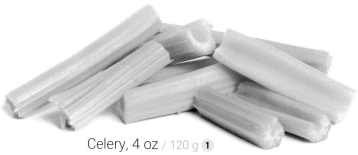

Celery, 4 oz / 120 g **1**

3 = Protein in grams.

Vital Snacks
Vegetables and dip *continued*

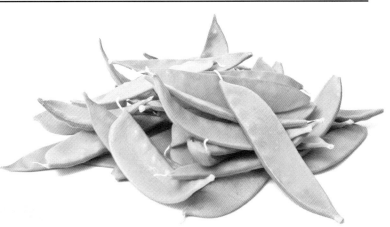

Snow peas, 1.5 cups, 6.7 oz / 200 g **3**

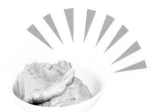

2 Tbsp
creamy dip **1**
fat free cream cheese **3**
or hummus **3**

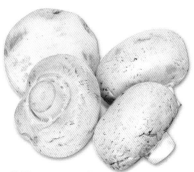

Mushrooms, 2.7 oz / 80 g **3**

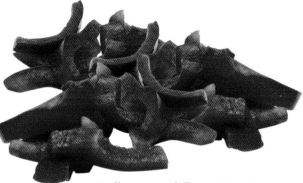

Bell pepper, 2.7 oz / 80 g **1**

Edamame beans, 1 cup in shell, 4.2 oz / 125 g **1**

3 = Protein in grams.

Vital Snacks
Dairy

Dairy snacks are a great idea for between meals because the protein keeps you feeling satisfied. Most low fat dairy snacks are low GI despite added sugar.

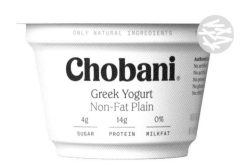

Yogurt, light or low fat plain,
6.7 oz / 200 g **15**

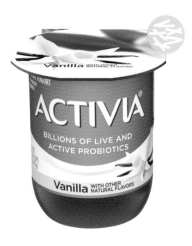

Yogurt, flavoured, low fat,
4 oz / 120 g **5**

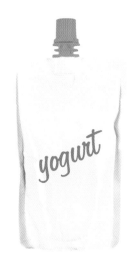

Yogurt pouch or tube,
2.3 oz / 70 g **3**

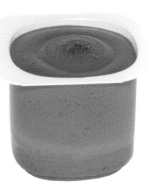

Low fat custard, mousse or pudding cups,
½ cup, 3.3 oz / 100 g **4**

3 = Protein in grams. = Contains probiotic bacteria.

Vital Snacks

Dairy *continued*

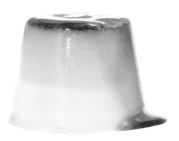

Creme Caramel / Spanish style custard
½ cup, 4 oz / 125 g **6.5**

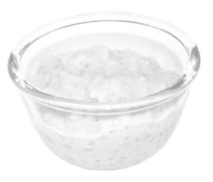

Low fat or sugar free pudding,
½ cup, 4 oz / 125 g **3**

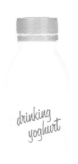

Drinking Yogurt,
3.3 fl oz / 100 ml **2**

^Reduced / low fat / skim milk,
6.7 oz / 200 ml **8**

Continued over ❯

3 = Protein in grams. ^ Refer to page 39 for 100 Calorie serves of plant based milks.

Vital Snacks

Dairy *continued*

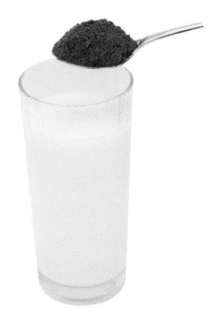

^Skim milk, 6.7 oz / 200 ml + 1 hpd tsp
sugar reduced Nesquik **9**

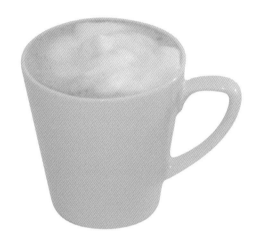

^Skinny Cappuccino or Flat White,
6.7 oz / 200 ml **6**

Triscuits, 2 +
1 slice cheese with 2% milk **8**

String Cheese, 2%,
2 x 20 g sticks, **7**

---

* Everyday criteria for milk, Yogurts + desserts per 100 Cal / 420 kJ **pack**
1. 3 g or less of fat
2. Low GI or 20 g or less of sugar (most dairy foods are low GI)

* Everyday criteria for cheeses per 100 Cal / 420 kJ **serve**
1. 6g or less of fat

---

3 = Protein in grams. ^ Refer to page 39 for 100 Calorie serves of plant based milks.

Vital Snacks
Higher Protein Choices

A higher protein choice at mid morning is a great idea for your morning snack. While any time of day is great, evidence suggests that protein is best distributed evenly throughout the day, and a higher protein morning snack can balance the amount consumed at breakfast with the larger intake that typically occurs in the evening.

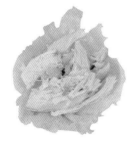

Chicken wrapped in lettuce, 2 oz / 60 g **16**

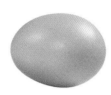

Boiled egg, 1 extra large **6**

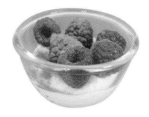

Raspberries, 6 with cottage cheese, ⅓ cup **11**

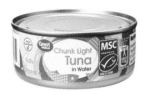

Tuna, 100 g **18**

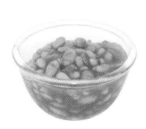

Baked Beans, 130 g **6**

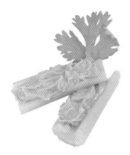

Celery sticks, with crunchy nut butter, 3 tsp **5**

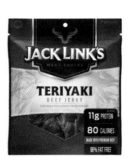

Just Jerky Beef Jerky, all flavours, 80 g **11**

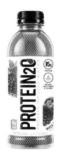

Protein infused water, 500 ml **15**

3 = Protein in grams.

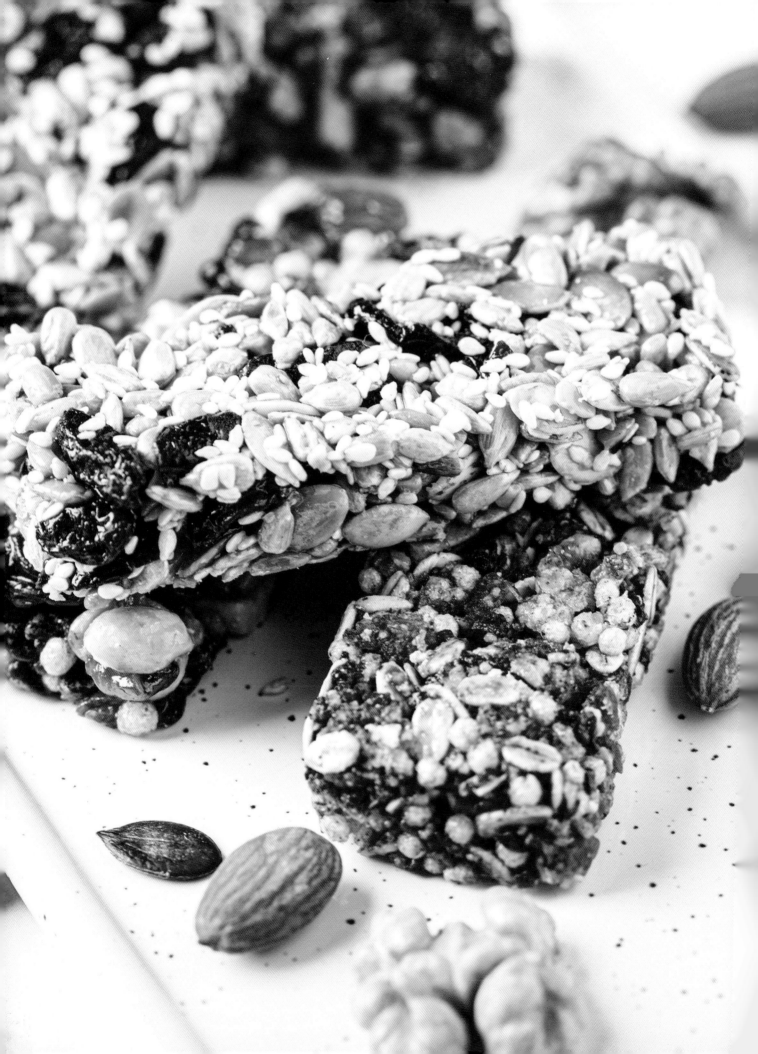

Occasional Snacks
Bars

Occasional snacks meet general healthy criteria and are portion controlled at 100 Cals. These snacks are not as high in the nutrients critical to health on a tightly restricted food intake. Focus intake around the vital snacks on a daily basis, and include these other healthy snacks a couple of times a week for variety and flexibility. Muesli bars can be a handy snack, but make sure they're made of healthy ingredients and only contain 100 Cals. Look for fruit and wholegrains with a smattering of nuts.

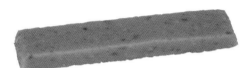

Fruit bar, 0.7 oz / 20 g **0**

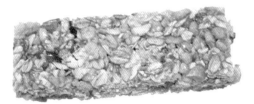

Granola bar, 1 oz / 35 g **2**

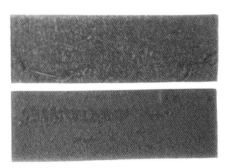

Fruit straps, 2 **0**

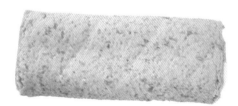

Baked Fruit Bar, 1.3 oz / 40 g **1**

---

* Everyday bar criteria

Approx 100 Cals / 420 kJ **per serve and 3 out of 4 of the following criteria:**
  1. 1 g or more of fibre
  2. Low GI or 5 g or less of sugar if no/ little fruit or

15 g or less sugar with significant fruit*
  3. 3.5 g or less fat if no nuts or 7.5 g or less fat with nuts.
  4. 1 g or less saturated fat.
  *significant fruit is considered to be 25% or more.

---

3 = Protein in grams.

Occasional Snacks (2/wk)
Frozen desserts

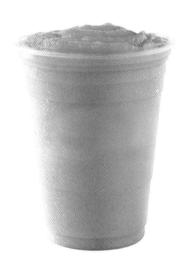

Frappucino Coffee flavour, no cream, 12 fl oz / 350 ml **4**

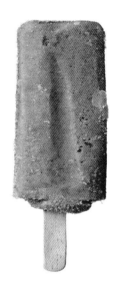

Milk ice, 2 oz / 60 g **2**

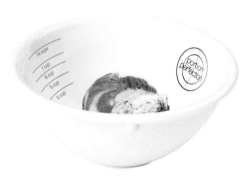

Light Ice cream, various brands, 1 scoop, 3.3 fl oz / 100 ml **2**

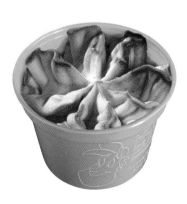

Frozen Yogurt, 1 scoop, 1.5 oz / 45 g **1**

3 = Protein in grams.

Occasional Snacks (2/wk)
Biscuits, cookies and crackers

Most biscuits and crackers are high GI however those with either wholegrains or fruit tend to be lower. Try low fat dips with healthy crackers.

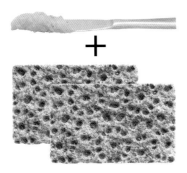

Low GI or grainy crackers, 2 large, + 2 tsp low fat dip **2**

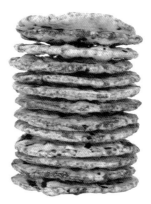

Wholegrain rice snacks, 13 **2**

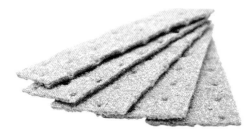

Thin rye crispread, 5, 0.8 oz / 25 g **3**

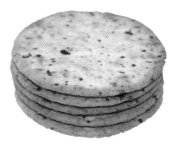

Low GI or grainy crackers, 5 small **3**

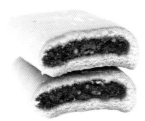

Fruit filled cookies, 2 **1**

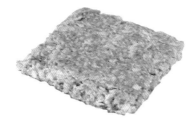

Muesli cookie, 1, 0.5 oz / 17 g **1**

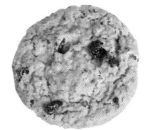

Raisin or oat cookie, 1 standard size, 0.8 oz / 25 g **1**

Everyday biscuit/cookie criteria* per 100 Cal / 420 kJ **serve**

1. 3 g or less of saturated fat
2. 200 mg or less of sodium
3. Low GI or 10% wholegrains or 25% or more of fruit

* Biscuits/Cookies should meet all criteria. Some products in this category do not declare data relevant to criteria 3, some professional judgements have been made.

---

3 = Protein in grams.

Occasional Snacks (2/wk)
Miscellaneous

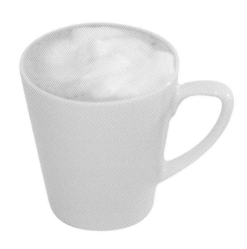

^Hot chocolate, low fat, 6.7 oz / 200 ml **9**

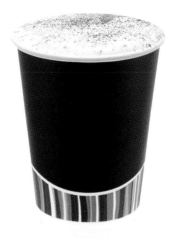

^Cappuccino or Flat White, fat free, 12 oz / 350 ml **9**

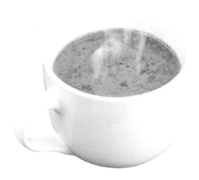

Instant soup, 6.7 oz / 200 ml **9**

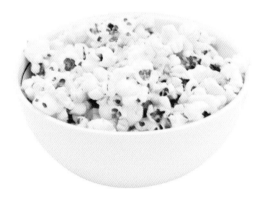

Popcorn, 1.5 cups **1**

3 = Protein in grams. ^ Refer to page 39 for 100 Calorie serves of plant based milks.

Occasional Snacks (2/wk)
Miscellaneous *continued*

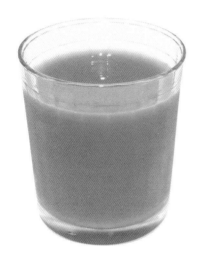

Vegetable juice, 10 fl oz / 300 ml **3**

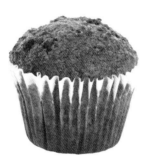

Mini bran muffin or dark fruit cake, 1 oz / 30 g **1**

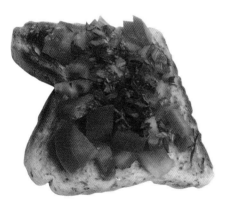

Toast with Tomato and Herbs, 1 Slice **3**

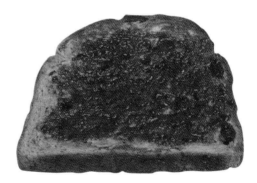

Raisin Toast with fruit spread, 1 slice **3**

Foods for this category have been chosen for their proximity to 100 Cals / 420 kJ per serve and either:
1. Real food ingredients
2. Low GI
3. Nutrient content

---

3 = Protein in grams.

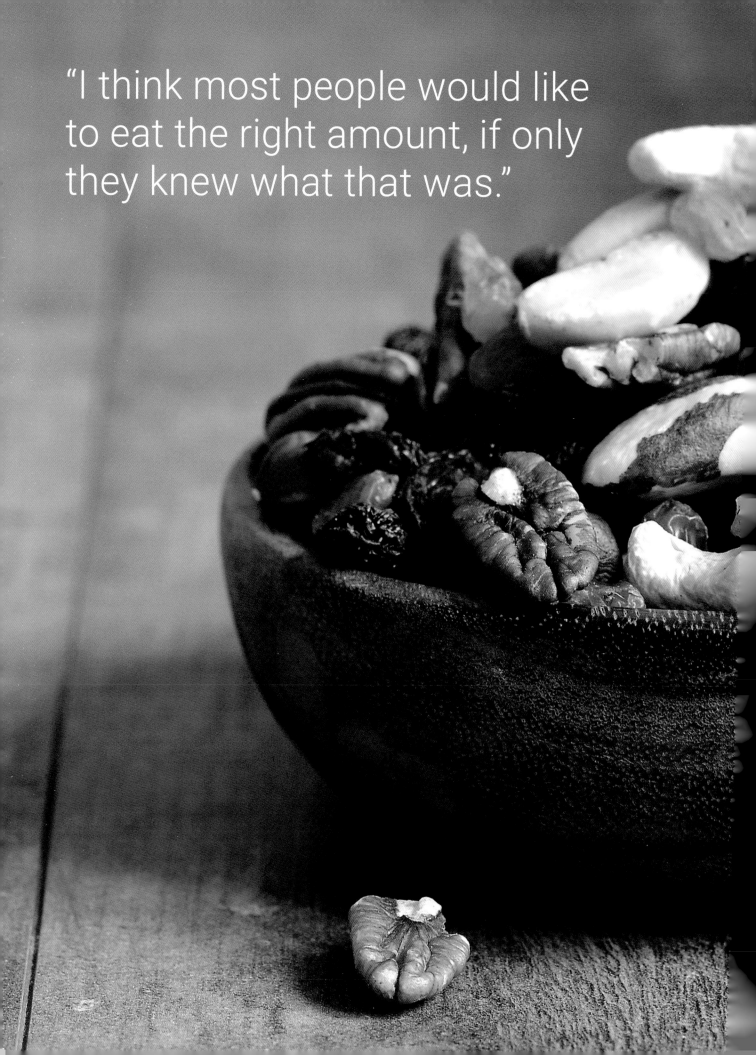

"I think most people would like to eat the right amount, if only they knew what that was."

appendices

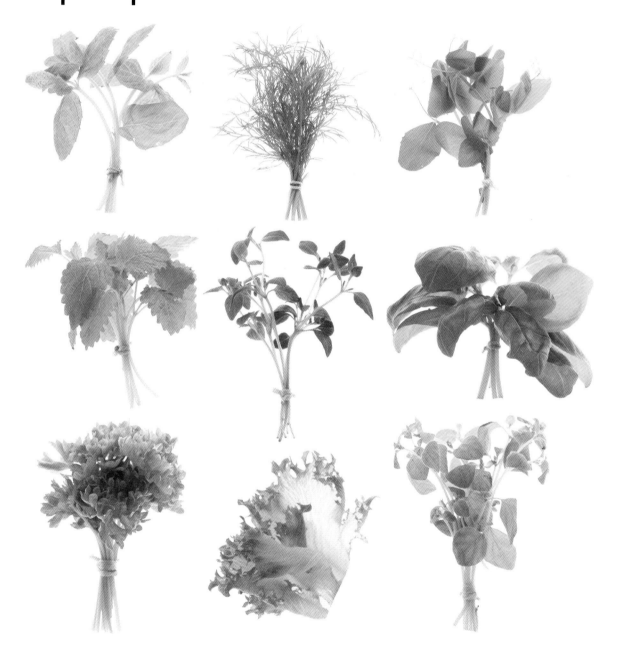

Appendix 1

Fruit = 50 Cals / 210 kJ

A small piece of fruit, weighing approximately 3.3 oz / 100 g equates to 50 Cals / 210 kJ. Larger serves of fruit weighing 6.7 oz / 200 g equate to 100 Cals / 420 kJ. Small pieces only are shown in this section – simply double the portion for a 100 Cal / 420 kJ Add On or an everyday snack.

Apple, 1 small, 3.3 oz / 100 g **0**

Apricots, 3, 3 oz / 90 g **1**

Dried apricots, 5, 1 oz / 30 g **1**

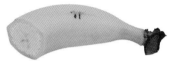
Banana, ½ medium, 2 oz / 60 g **1**

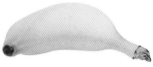
Lady-finger banana, 2 oz / 60 g **1**

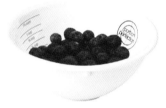
Blueberries, ½ cup, 2.5 oz / 75 g **0**

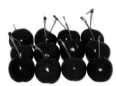
Cherries, 12 med, 2.5 oz / 72 g **1**

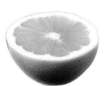
Grapefruit, 1 med, 6.7 oz / 200 g **1**

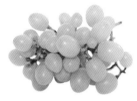
Grapes, small bunch, 3.3 oz / 100 g **1**

Kiwi fruit, med, 3.3 oz / 100 g **1**

Mandarin, med, 4 oz / 120 g **1**

Mango, ½ small, 3.3 oz / 100 g **2**

Nectarine, med, 4 oz / 120 g **2**

Orange, small, 5 oz / 150 g **1**

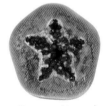
Papaya, ½ med, 5 oz / 150 g **1**

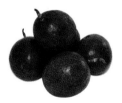
Passionfruit, 4, 5 oz / 150 g **2**

Peach, med, 4 oz / 120 g **1**

Pear, small, 4 oz / 120 g **0**

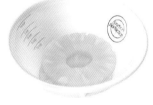
Pineapple, 2 slices, 3.3 oz / 100 g **1**

Plums, 2 med, 4 oz / 120 g **1**

Prunes, 5 small, 1 oz / 25 g **1**

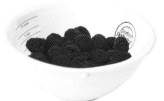
Raspberries, ¾ cup, 2.5 oz / 75 g **1**

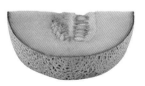
Rockmelon / Cantaloupe, 4.7 oz / 140 g **1**

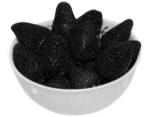
Strawberries, 1½ cups, 8.3 oz / 250 g **4**

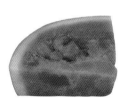
Watermelon, 8.3 oz / 250 g **1**

3 = Protein in grams.

Fruit *continued*

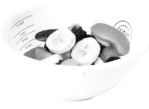
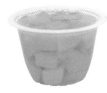

Dried fruit, 1.5 Tbsp,
0.7 oz / 20 g **0**

Fruit salad, ½ cup,
3.3 oz / 100 g **1**

Canned fruit, ½ cup,
4.7 oz / 140 g **0**

If you prefer some more exotic fruit, check the amount for a 50 Cal / 210 kJ serve via **Calorieking** (USA & Aust) or
My Fitness Pal (UK) and record it here.

---

3 = Protein in grams.

Appendix 2

Add ons = 100 Cals / 420 kJ

"Add ons" are foods that easily add to meals and contain approximately 100 Cals / 420 kJ. Use this section to develop your knowledge so you'll be able to look at a meal served in a café and easily 'count up' the approximate Calories so you know where to stop. Any choice from the snack list could appear here, however we have shown representative images for simplicity.

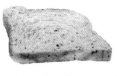
Bread, 1 slice (no spread), 1 oz / 30 g **3**

Fruit, large, 1 piece **2**

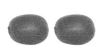
Fruit, small, 2 pieces **2**

Avocado, ¹/₃, 2 oz / 60 g **1**

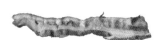
Bacon, 2 short cut or 1 full rasher, 1.7 oz / 50 g **15**

Cheese, full fat, 0.7 oz / 20 g **5**

Cheese, 50% less fat, 2 slices, 1.3 oz / 40 g **14**

Parmesan cheese, 0.7 oz / 20 g **8**

Grated cheese, 0.7 oz / 20 g **5**

Egg, fried, 1 large, 1.9 oz / 55 g **8**

Eggs, 2 small, 2.7 oz / 80 g **10**

Nuts, 0.7 oz / 20 g **4**

Mayonnaise, 3 tsp **1**

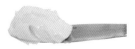
Butter / marg, 3 tsp **1**

Instant soup, various brands **1**

Olives, 10, 3.3 oz / 100 g **1**

Tuna, salmon or chicken, 1 small can, 3.7 oz / 110 g **20**

Oil, 2 tsp **0**

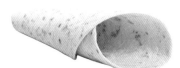
Tortilla, 1 small, 1 oz / 30 g **4**

Spaghetti, 1 can, 4.3 oz / 130 g **2**

Baked beans, 4.3 oz / 130 g **6**

Corn, kernels or creamed, 3.3 oz / 100 g **3**

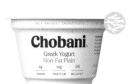
Yogurt, light or low fat plain, 6.7 oz / 200 g **15**

Yogurt, flavoured, low fat, 4 oz / 120 g **4**

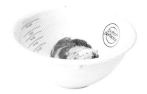
Light Ice cream, various brands, 1 scoop, 3.3 fl oz / 100 ml **2**

Low fat custard, mousse or pudding cups, ½ cup, 3.3 oz / 100 g **4**

3 = Protein in grams. ⬭ = Contains probiotic bacteria.

Appendix 2

Add ons *continued*

Occasional Add Ons

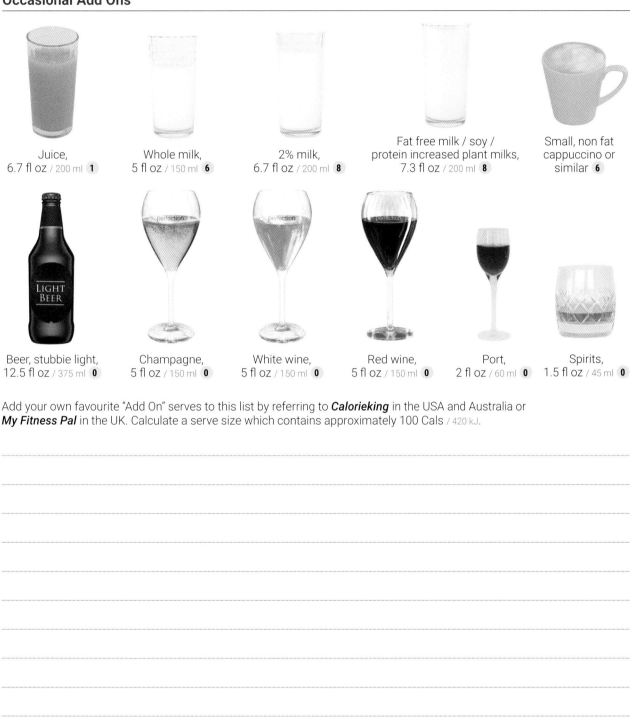

Juice,
6.7 fl oz / 200 ml **1**

Whole milk,
5 fl oz / 150 ml **6**

2% milk,
6.7 fl oz / 200 ml **8**

Fat free milk / soy /
protein increased plant milks,
7.3 fl oz / 200 ml **8**

Small, non fat
cappuccino or
similar **6**

Beer, stubbie light,
12.5 fl oz / 375 ml **0**

Champagne,
5 fl oz / 150 ml **0**

White wine,
5 fl oz / 150 ml **0**

Red wine,
5 fl oz / 150 ml **0**

Port,
2 fl oz / 60 ml **0**

Spirits,
1.5 fl oz / 45 ml **0**

Add your own favourite "Add On" serves to this list by referring to **Calorieking** in the USA and Australia or
My Fitness Pal in the UK. Calculate a serve size which contains approximately 100 Cals / 420 kJ.

3 = Protein in grams.

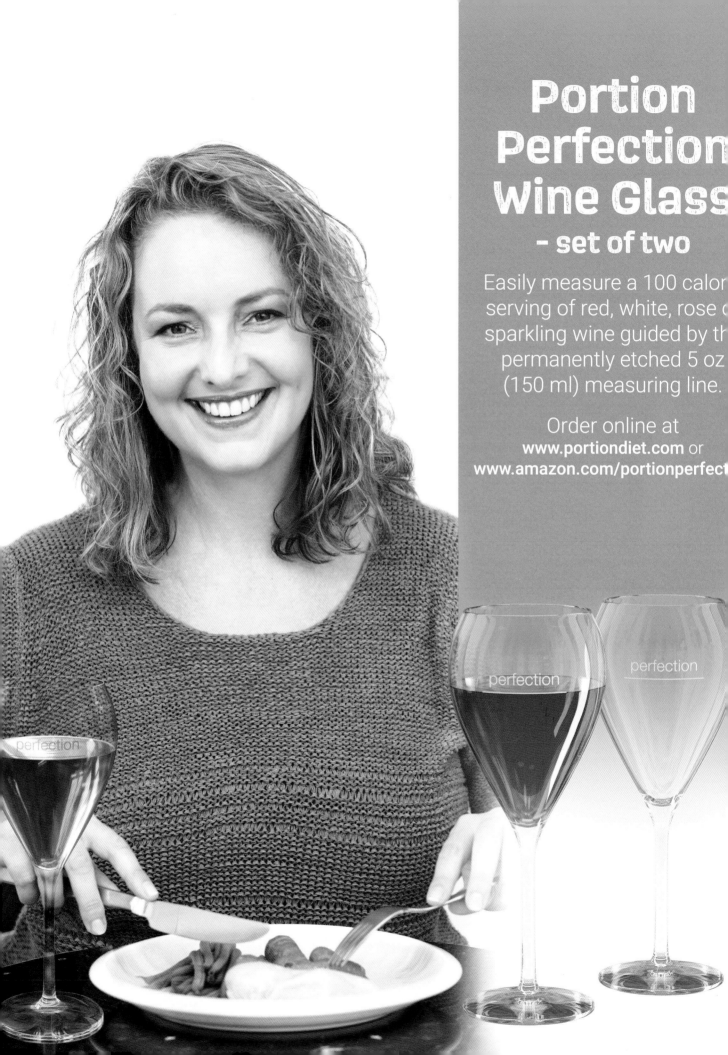

Portion Perfection Wine Glass
– set of two

Easily measure a 100 calor
serving of red, white, rose o
sparkling wine guided by th
permanently etched 5 oz
(150 ml) measuring line.

Order online at
www.portiondiet.com or
www.amazon.com/portionperfect

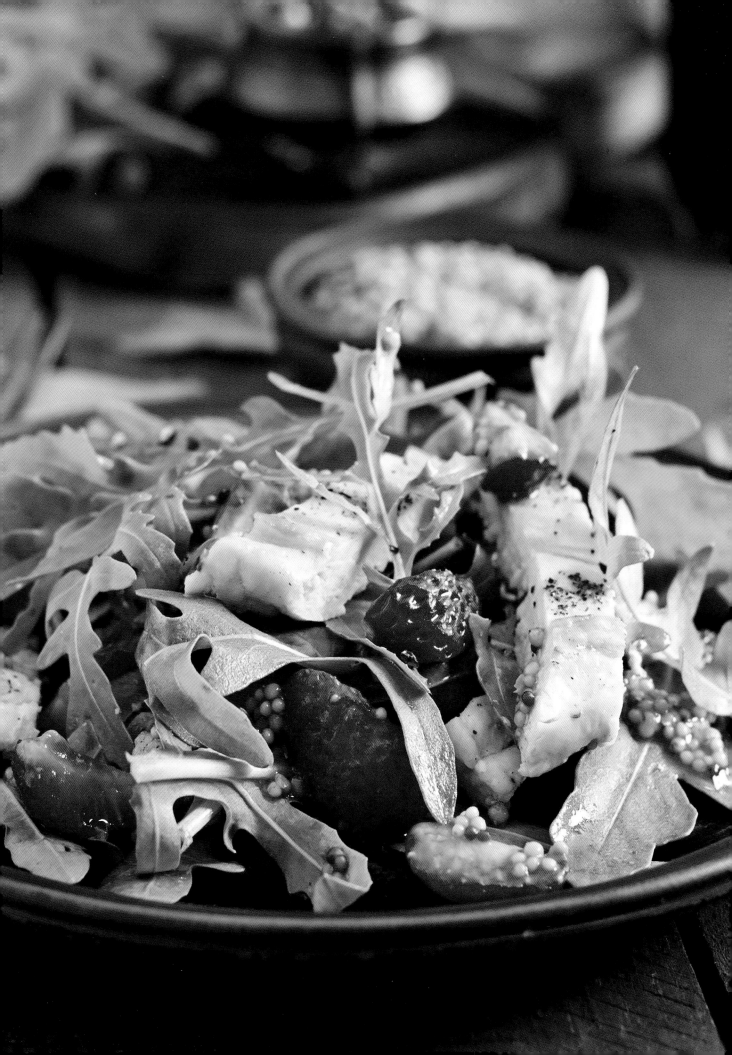

Appendix 3

Free Foods = <20 Cals / <84 kJ

'Free foods' refer to foods that are very low in Calories, contributing 20 Cals / 84 kJ or less in a specified serve. It is safe to add one of these in the amount shown to any meal. Water and mineral water can be added freely, and you can consider a cupful of salad or free vegetables as a 'free food' serve.

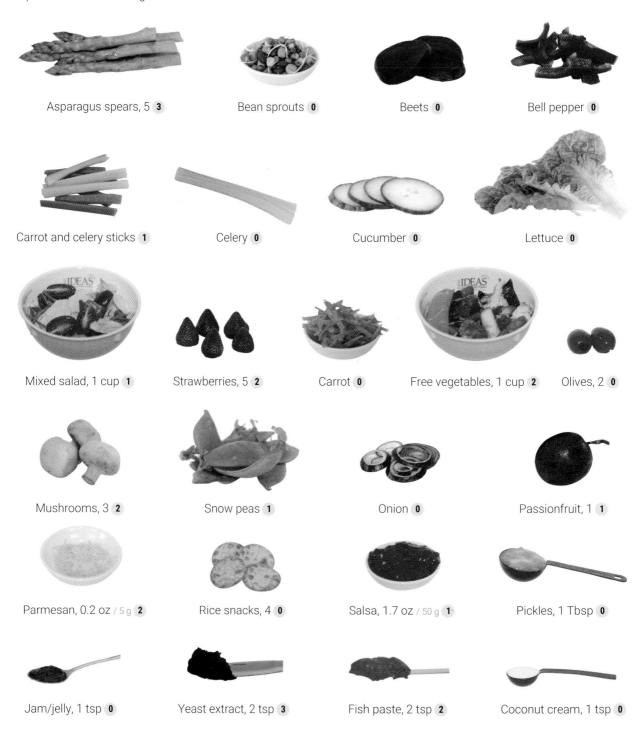

Asparagus spears, 5 **3**

Bean sprouts **0**

Beets **0**

Bell pepper **0**

Carrot and celery sticks **1**

Celery **0**

Cucumber **0**

Lettuce **0**

Mixed salad, 1 cup **1**

Strawberries, 5 **2**

Carrot **0**

Free vegetables, 1 cup **2**

Olives, 2 **0**

Mushrooms, 3 **2**

Snow peas **1**

Onion **0**

Passionfruit, 1 **1**

Parmesan, 0.2 oz / 5 g **2**

Rice snacks, 4 **0**

Salsa, 1.7 oz / 50 g **1**

Pickles, 1 Tbsp **0**

Jam/jelly, 1 tsp **0**

Yeast extract, 2 tsp **3**

Fish paste, 2 tsp **2**

Coconut cream, 1 tsp **0**

3 = Protein in grams.

Appendix 3

Free Foods *continued*

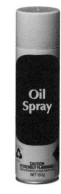

Kraft Free Mayo,
1 Tbsp, 0.7 oz / 20 g **0**

Sour cream,
1 tsp **0**

Low fat sauce
(eg tomato), 1 Tbsp **0**

High fat sauce
(eg bearnaise), 1 tsp **0**

Spray oil
(2 second spray) **0**

Sugar cube, 1 **0**

Chocolate, 1 square **0**

Cough drop, 1 **0**

Chewing gum,
all types, 4 pieces **0**

Animal Crackers, 2 **0**

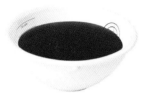

Clear soup / broth, 1 cup **1**

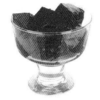

Sugar free Jello, 1 cup **1**

Milk, all types,
1 fl oz / 30 ml **1**

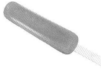

Sugar free popsicle,
1 stick, 1.6 fl oz / 48 ml **0**

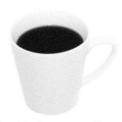

Herbal or black tea or coffee with
1 tsp sugar **0** or 1 fl oz / 30 ml milk **1**

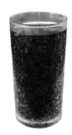

Diet soda,
8 fl oz / 250 ml **1**

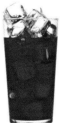

Crystal Light powdered drink
mix, 1 glass, 8 fl oz / 250ml **0**

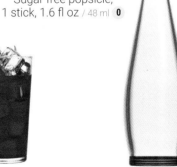

Water or Mineral water
(any time) **0**

Add your own favourite "Free Foods" serves to this list by referring to **Calorieking** in the USA and Australia or
My Fitness Pal in the UK. Calculate a serve size which contains approximately 20 Cals / 84 kJ or less.

3 = Protein in grams.

Anna's quick and easy chickpea and vegetable casserole

While the list of ingredients looks long, many are pantry staples and the method is straightforward!

Ingredients

½ brown onion

1 carrot, peeled and chopped

2 cloves garlic, crushed

2cm piece ginger, finely grated

1 Tbsp olive oil

1 tsp ground coriander (cilantro)

½ tsp ground cumin

½ tsp ground turmeric

½ tsp red chilli flakes

½ cube salt-reduced stock cube made up in 10 fl oz / 300 ml boiling water

13.3 oz / 400 g tin crushed (or diced) Italian tomatoes

13.3 oz / 400 g tin no added salt chickpeas

1 cup broccoli florets

1 cup coriander (cilantro) leaves, picked

1 squeeze fresh lemon juice

Fresh cracked pepper, to taste

Method

1. Heat oil in a heavy based pan over medium heat and sauté onion until becoming translucent.

2. Add in carrot, garlic and ginger. Cook, stirring for 2 minutes.

3. Add dried spices and stir until aromatic (about 1-2 minutes).

4. Add stock, chickpeas tomato, stirring. Bring to the boil and reduce heat to a simmer. Simmer for 15 minutes or until carrot and onion is soft.

5. Add broccoli and cauliflower florets, stirring to cover in sauces. Cover and allow to cook, stirring occasionally, for 5 minutes or until vegetables are cooked to your liking.

6. Add in coriander (cilantro), fresh lemon juice and season with cracked pepper. Remove from the heat and stir.

7. Serve 1 cup portions. Any leftovers freeze well. If you are a diabetic and need additional carbohydrates, serve with a small amount of couscous on the side.

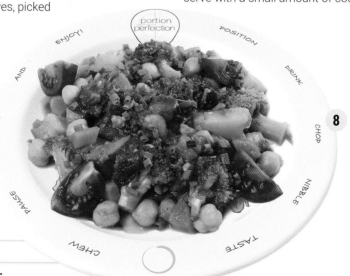

Makes 4 x 1 cup serves			
Nutritional Information per serve:			
Energy	200 Cals / 840 kJ	Carbohydrate	18.6 g
Protein	8.5 g	Sugars	5 g
Fat	7 g	Fibre	7.6 g
Saturated Fat	1 g	Sodium	2.7 mg

3 = Protein in grams.

Appendix 5
My meal plan

Breakfast

Mid morning snack

Lunch

Mid afternoon snack

Dinner

Supper

Appendix 5
Menu Planner

Use this planner to plan your weeks food intake. Use any of the great cookbooks from **www.greatideas.net.au** or **www.portiondiet.com** to keep things interesting. Put all the ingredients for the meals straight onto the shopping list so you have every fiddly little herb and spice to make the meals perfect.

	BREAKFAST	LUNCH	DINNER	SNACKS
MONDAY				
TUESDAY				
WEDNESDAY				
THURSDAY				
FRIDAY				
SATURDAY				
SUNDAY				

Appendix 5
Shopping List

Groceries

Meat, seafood and poultry

Fruit & Vegetables

Dairy

Other

A final word...

I think legislation should be introduced that requires that the information on the nutrition panel relates to a realistic serving size.

I think there needs to be support for companies who package foods in serving sizes that match Calorie needs.

I'd like to see the 'party food' section of the supermarket move into a separate shop so that we are making a conscious decision to go and purchase these foods, rather than having them leap into our trolleys while doing the groceries. I think if we only actually ate cakes and lollies and crisps and drank soda pop and alcohol at parties, we wouldn't be in this mess. Instead we're led to believe that a king sized chocolate bar is an acceptable purchase while filling up with gas. In fact the attendants suggestive-sell chocolate bars in some gas stations.

We are now seeing the Calorie or kiloJoule contents displayed in food outlets in some places around the world and more are following. Data from New York proves that when you see that the muffin you like to eat with your coffee contains 500 or 600 Calories / 2100 or 2520 kJ it is less appealing, resulting in an average decrease in calorie intake by 6% for every purchase made.

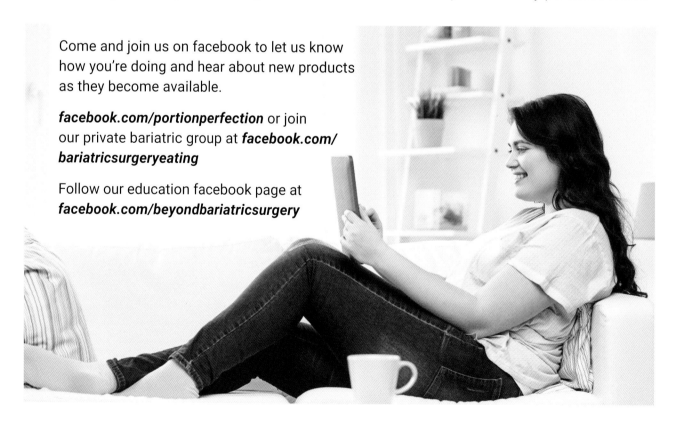

Come and join us on facebook to let us know how you're doing and hear about new products as they become available.

facebook.com/portionperfection or join our private bariatric group at *facebook.com/ bariatricsurgeryeating*

Follow our education facebook page at *facebook.com/beyondbariatricsurgery*

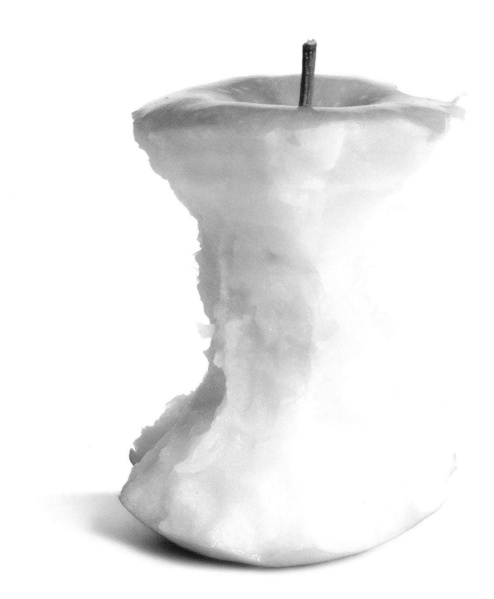

Bariatric Products

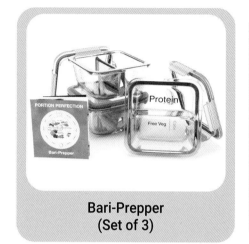

Bari-Prepper
(Set of 3)

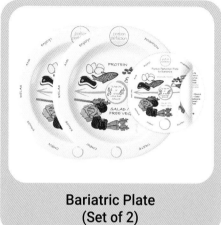

Bariatric Plate
(Set of 2)

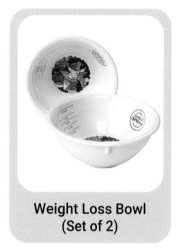

Weight Loss Bowl
(Set of 2)

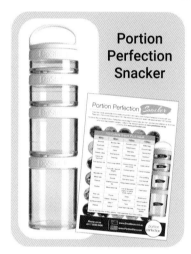

Portion Perfection Snacker

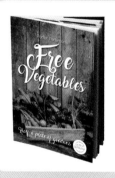
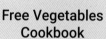

Free Vegetables Cookbook

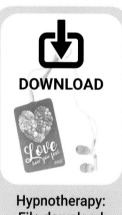

DOWNLOAD

Hypnotherapy: File download

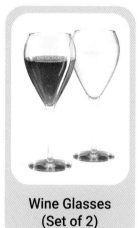

Wine Glasses
(Set of 2)

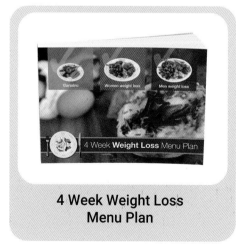

4 Week Weight Loss Menu Plan

NEW PRODUCT

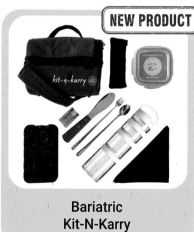

Bariatric Kit-N-Karry

NEW PRODUCT

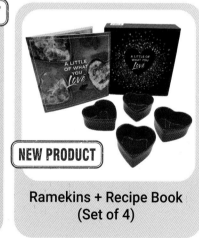

Ramekins + Recipe Book
(Set of 4)

Portion Perfection Products

The purple version of Portion Perfection contains plans for men, women and children and a larger plate than the bariatric version. The bowls, snack bible and hypnotherapy apply to everyone.

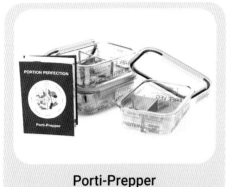

**Porti-Prepper
(Set of 3)**

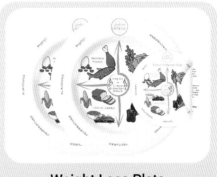

**Weight Loss Plate
(Set of 2)**

**Weight Loss Bowl
(Set of 2)**

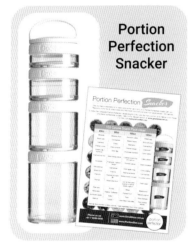

**Portion
Perfection
Snacker**

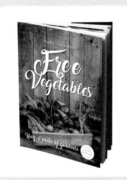

**Free Vegetables
Cookbook**

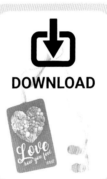

DOWNLOAD

**Hypnotherapy:
File download**

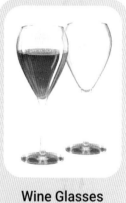

**Wine Glasses
(Set of 2)**

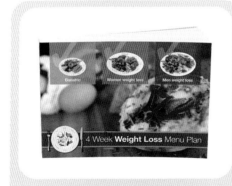

**4 Week Weight Loss
Menu Plan**

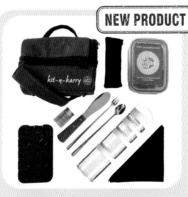

NEW PRODUCT

**Weight Loss
Kit-N-Karry**

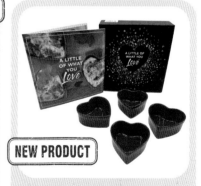

NEW PRODUCT

**Ramekins + Recipe Book
(Set of 4)**

Order online at **www.portiondiet.com** or **www.amazon.com/portionperfection**
Portion Perfection

Portions to go with
kit-ŋ-karry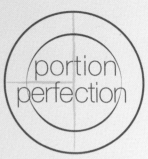

Take your meal prep container, snacks and all the tools you need with you, in our new Kit-n-Karry lunch bag.

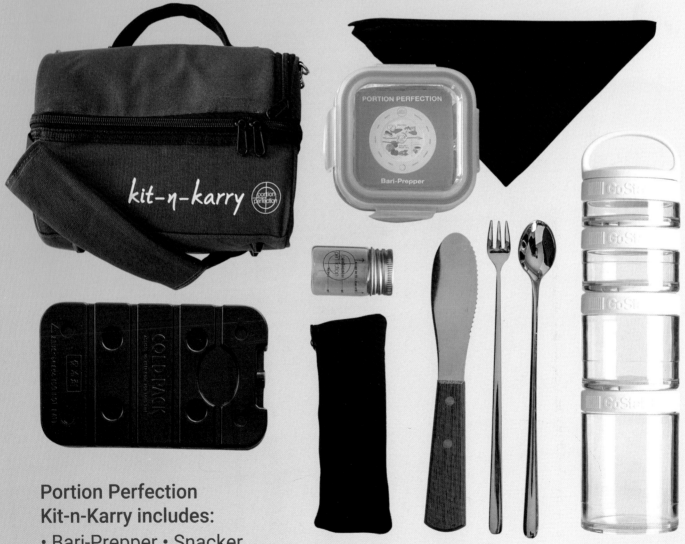

**Portion Perfection
Kit-n-Karry includes:**
- Bari-Prepper • Snacker
- Portion Control Fork & Spoon
- Cutlery pouch • Spreader/Spatula
- Sauce Container • Fabric Napkin • Ice Brick

*There's also one
for weight loss*